wise guys

A boy's guide to life

Sharon Witt

Wiseguys® – A Boy's Guide to Life

First printed August 2015
Second reprint February 2017
Third reprint October 2020
Fourth reprint February 2021
Fifth reprint July 2022
Sixth reprint November 2022
Seventh reprint February 2023
Eighth reprint May 2023
Ninth reprint July 2023
Tenth reprint August 2023
Eleventh reprint August 2024
Twelfth reprint September 2024
Thirteenth reprint January 2025
Fourteenth reprint January 2026

Published by Collective Wisdom Publications Pty Ltd
PO Box 150
Mt Evelyn Victoria 3796

National Library of Australia Cataloguing-in-Publication entry.

Creator:	Witt, Sharon, 1970- author.
Title:	Wiseguys : a boy's guide to life / Sharon Witt.
ISBN:	9780987277091 (paperback)
Series:	Witt, Sharon, 1970- Wiseguys ; volume 1.
Target Audience:	For primary school age.
Subjects:	Boys–Life skills guides.
	Boys–Conduct of life.

Dewey Number: 646.7

Design and cartoons: Ivan Smith, Communiqué Graphics, Lilydale
Printed by OBH Print

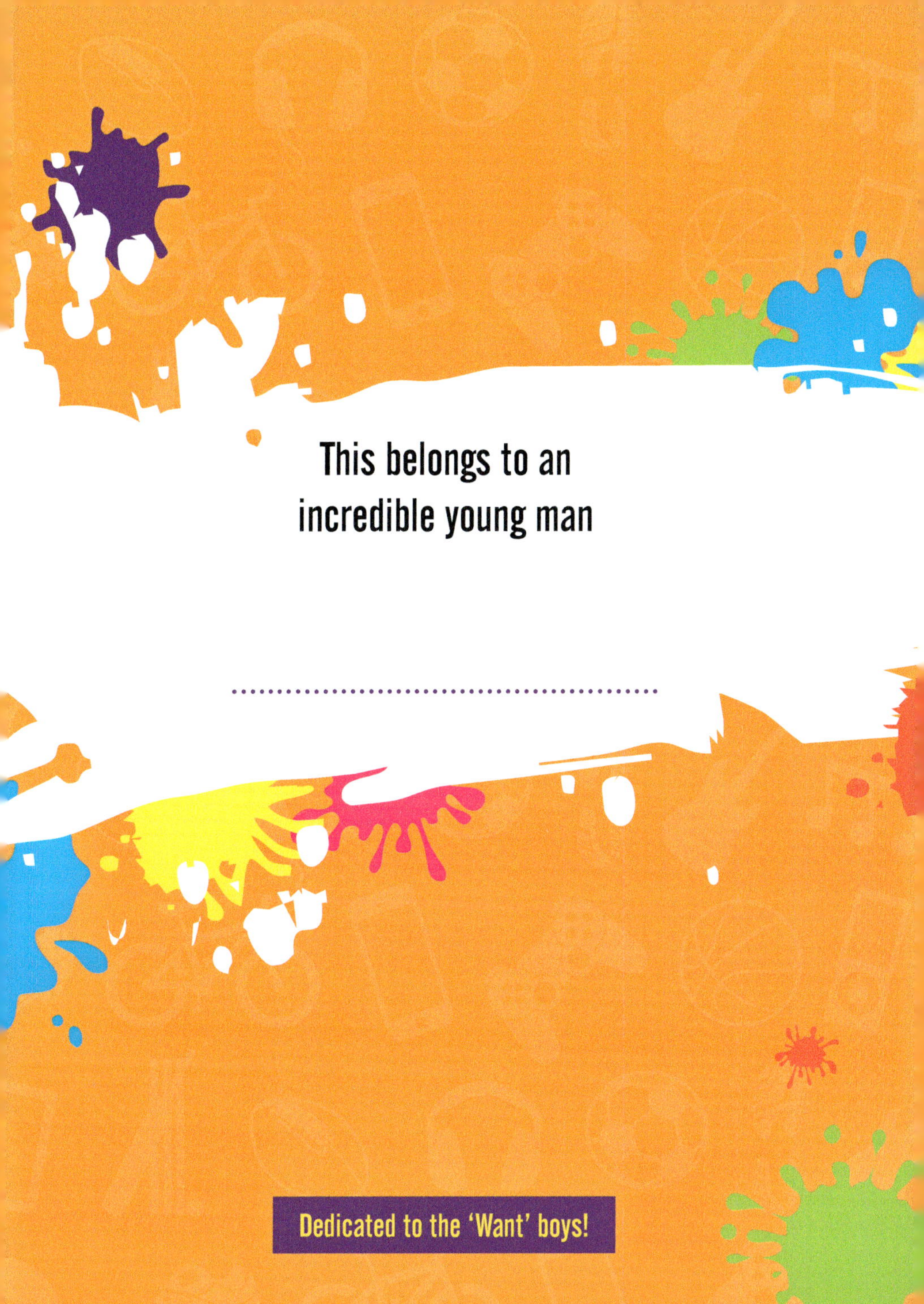
This belongs to an
incredible young man
Dedicated to the 'Want' boys!

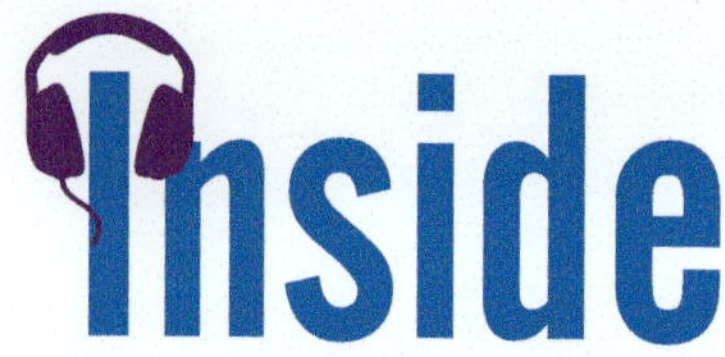

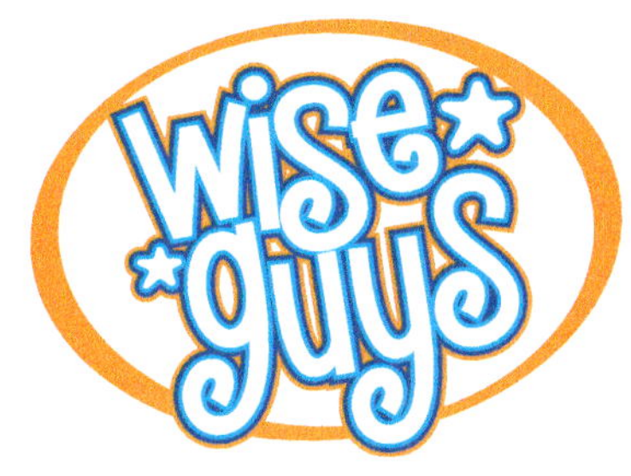

5 BULLYING

6 FEARS AND ANXIETIES

7 THE INTERNET AND SOCIAL MEDIA

8 MAKING MISTAKES

9 THINK POSITIVELY

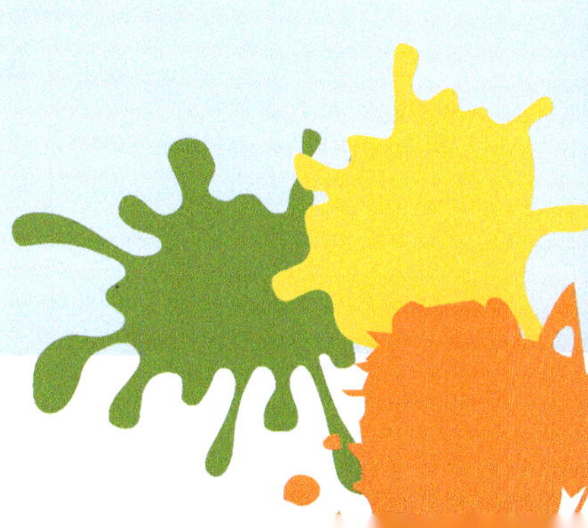

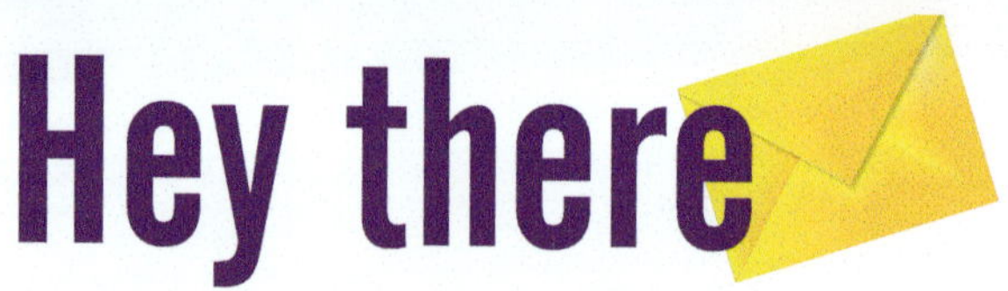

Hey there

...a message from me

Thanks for reading WISEGUYS – well, at least the first sentence, which makes me think you may be interested to see what's inside.

So why have I written this book? Actually, I wasn't planning to write a guide to growing up for guys. I write mostly for younger teens and older girls, sharing stories and advice to live happier, healthier, fulfilling lives. The sorts of things I normally write about are topics that range from hair to friendship hassles, and even hormones. What happened though, was a big surprise. After I'd finished writing another guide for girls, I got SO many requests to write a book for boys like yourself. Readers were telling me that they wanted something that helped guys — their sons, brothers, grandsons — to be their best in life.

So here it is, in your hands now. I hope that wherever you find yourself right now, and whatever you may be going through, the stories and advice in this book will help.

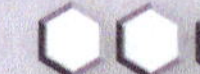

friends

bullies

problems

hormones

You may be thinking right now, 'Well, I'm not really a reader, so why bother?' Well, the GREAT news is, I've included a variety of helpful information to make it interesting and fun, clear, and easy to pick up and put down. As you turn each page, you'll see lots of quotes, funny stories and cartoons too. You pick what interests you the most.

For example, if you're having problems at school with friendships or even going through bullying, go straight to the section that talks about making friends or being a better friend. Or turn to the pages that will give you strategies and ideas to cope with bullying.

help!

I hope you enjoy reading it, and remember that you are NEVER alone!

You are incredible!

HAPPY READING.

Sharon

BE YOUR BEST

Where you are at!

In life, you will find that you have many different experiences. Some will be amazing, fun and unforgettable. Others will be ones you won't enjoy and prefer to forget. But everything you go through will help build your CHARACTER.

There may be pain, and often lessons to learn.

Some lessons and experiences will pass in moments, others may last whole seasons — slower to resolve, and more complex.

Some of those seasons might seem a little scary, such as starting school for the first time, or moving house, even shifting to new cities. But there are things you can do to help prepare for the changes ahead.

That's a big reason why I wrote this book. In your hands are words to help guide you through life and be better prepared for the twists and turns ahead.

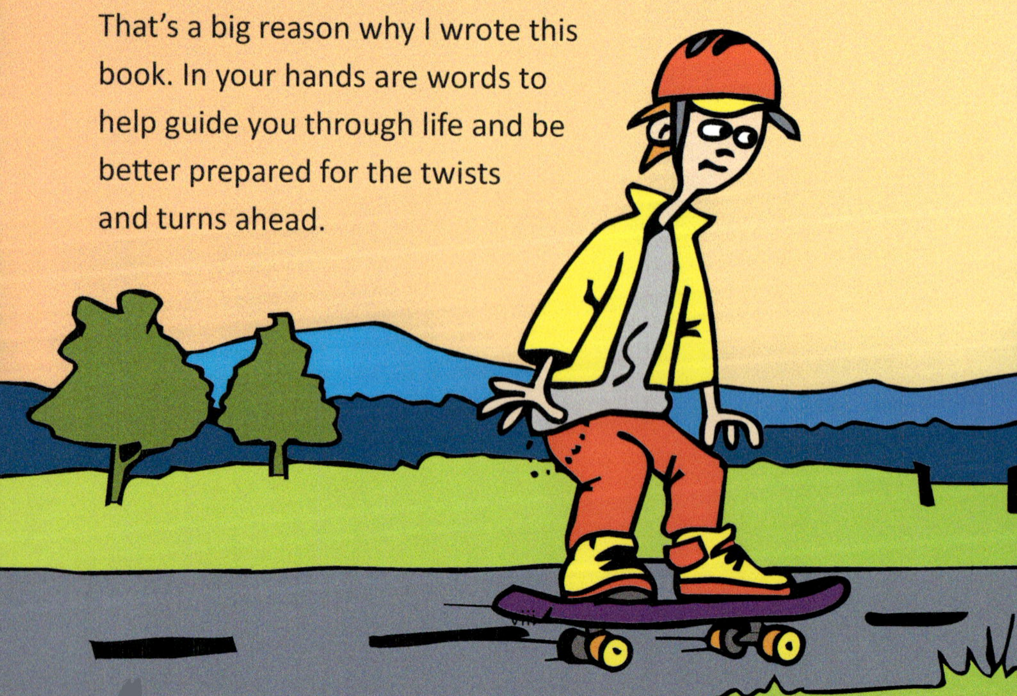

– Times and seasons

...this time will pass

Just remember, no season lasts forever. If you are in primary school now, for example, that is only for a time. Before you know it, you will be moving on up to high school. Or if you are having trouble with your mates today, you need to know that it won't last forever. Once you work through your problems with friends, or make choices to form new friendships, you will look back on the situation and hopefully come away with valuable lessons.

Wherever you are right now, you are not alone. You have wonderful people around you who will listen to what you have to say, and have words to help you in your journey. And you will grow to be a strong, incredible and awesome young man who will make a HUGE difference in this world.

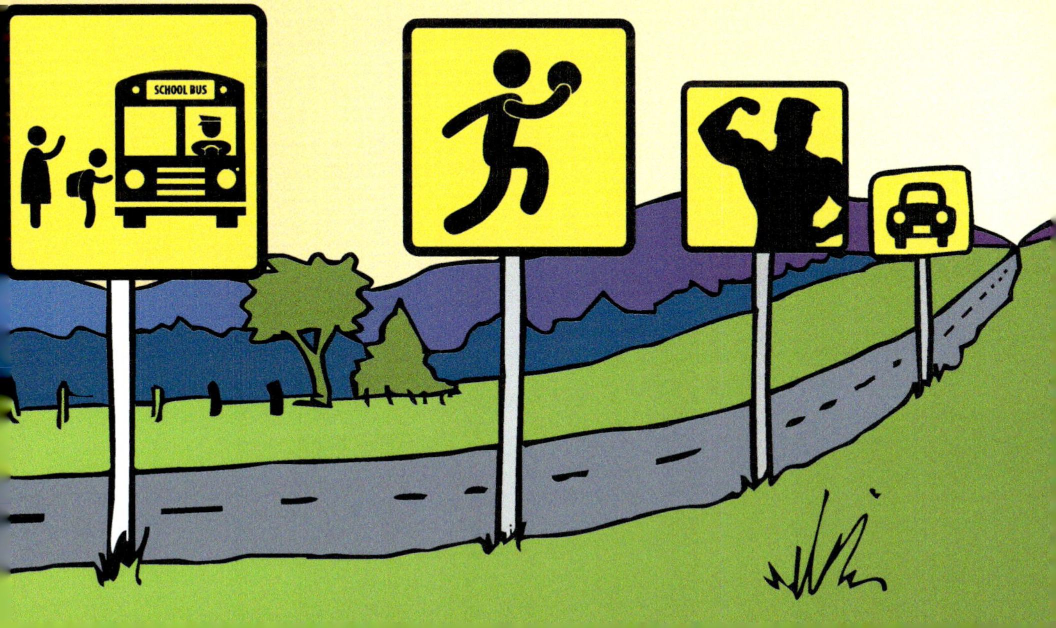

Seasons

Moving house

Moving schools

Starting school

Changing friendship groups

Family changes

A new addition to the family

Starting High School

Beginning a new sport or interest

New friends

Moving cities

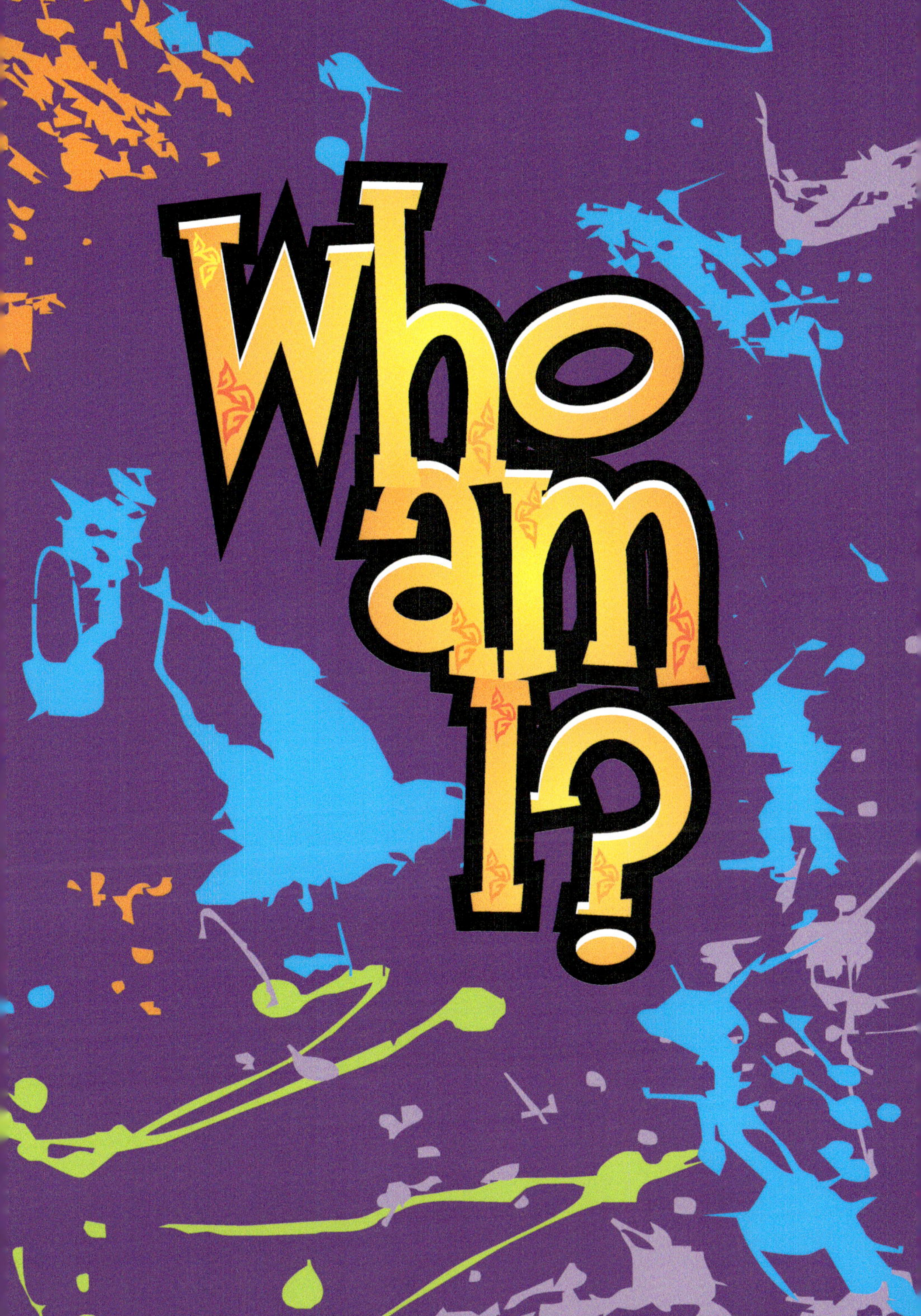
Who am I?

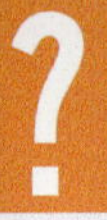

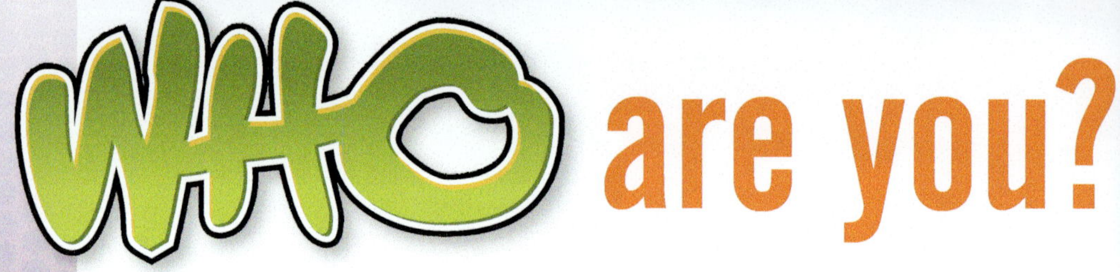

Who are you?

Who you are matters...

We have all been created as unique and valuable people, each with gifts and talents to bring to the world.

You, yes YOU, are a GIFT to the world.

You may not think that right at the moment, but trust me, you have all that you need within to make a difference to this planet.

Don't compare yourself

It is too easy to compare ourselves with others, thinking that their talents are worth more than anything we have to give. One day, while riding your bike with some mates, you may notice a guy who can do the most amazing jumps. He makes it all seem effortless.

'He is so talented,' you say to yourself. 'I just wish I could ride and do jumps like that.'

> 'Be yourself! Everyone else is already taken.'
> Oscar Wilde

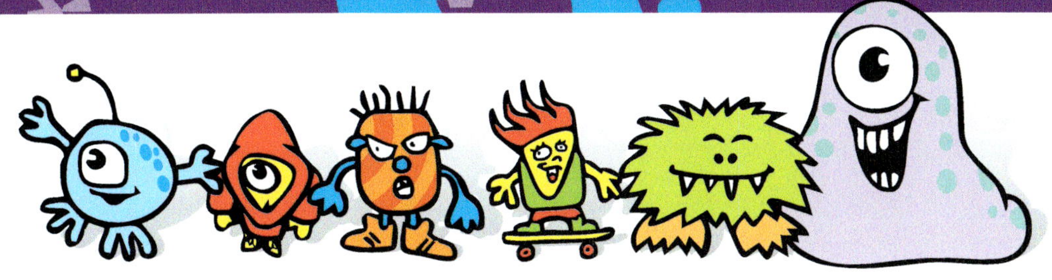

Or perhaps you hear your mate play a guitar and you think, 'Wow! That is very cool.' You just wish you could get up on stage and play an instrument with the confidence you see in him.

But here's the thing:
YOU have your gifts and
talents that are UNIQUE
to you.

Maybe you are a writer, able to use your imagination to create wonderful stories. Or perhaps you are gifted in sports, you are a brilliant runner, or score goals in a team.

You may be an incredible leader. Whenever you are called to form a group for a school project, you help others share their ideas and opinions, leading the way forward.

Concentrate on the things YOU are good at: the talents and gifts that YOU have been blessed with.

If we spend time focusing on what others are doing, we will deny them the chance to experience our gifts.

Your gifts & talents

Capable Caring Kind

Artistic Creative with writing

Confident Democratic

Capable leader Confident public speaker

Good mate Honest

Determined Loyal Creative

Intelligent Sporty Thoughtful

Loving Generous Spirited

Faithful Playful Resourceful

Musical Flexible

** If you don't know what any of these words mean, make sure you look them up in a dictionary.*

What's in your hand?

Try asking yourself today this question:
'What is in MY hand?'

What talents and strengths do you know you have that could help others around you? For examples of these, take another look at the words on the previous page.

Try and think of FIVE different talents or strengths you have and write them in the hand below.

RECORD

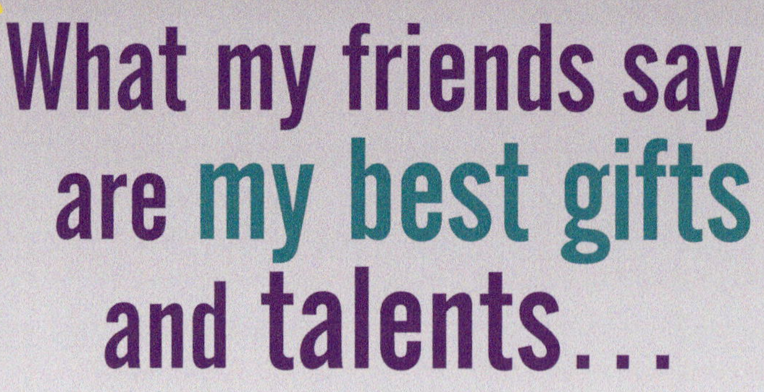

What my friends say are my best gifts and talents...

Interview one of your mates or family members to find out FIVE strengths or gifts that you have. Write them in the opened gifts below. It may be that the person you ask sees something you haven't identified in yourself.

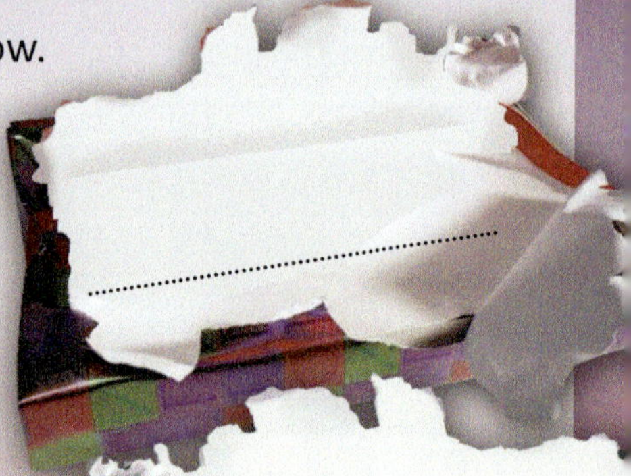

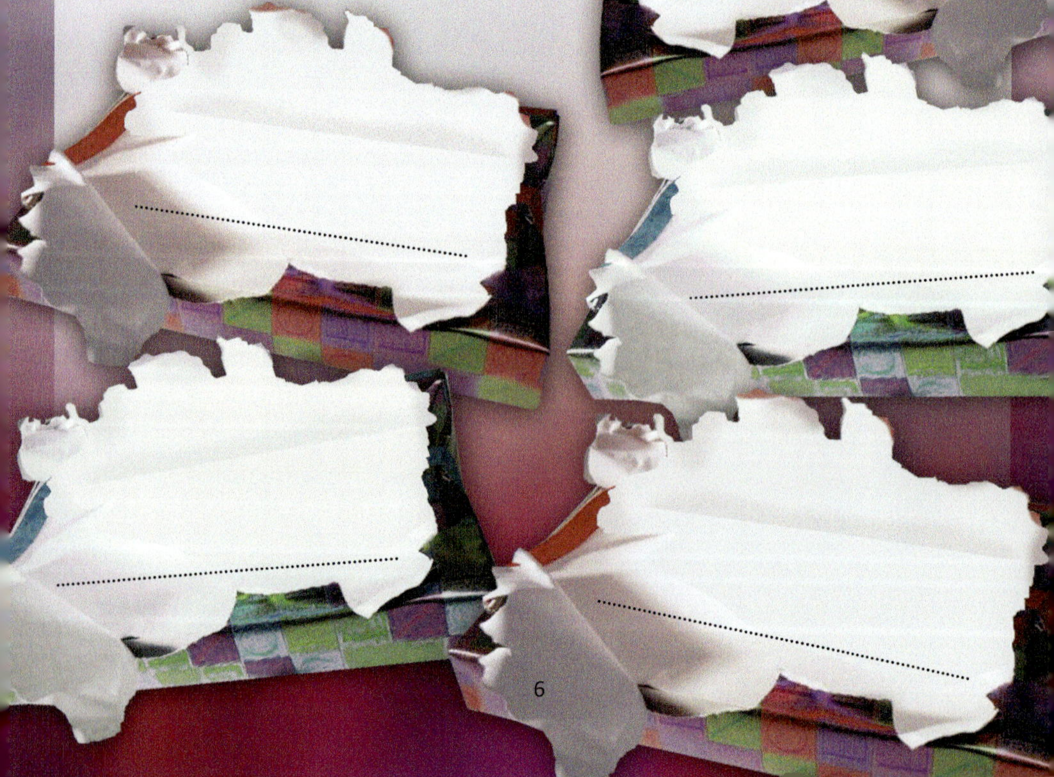

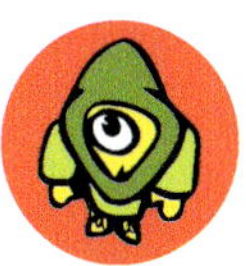

Matthew, aged 10

'I am good at bike riding, swimming, running, soccer and down ball. I can juggle and balance on a big ball at circus school. I love Minecraft.[1] I can ski on two skis, kneeboard, and love having fun on the biscuit[2] behind our boat with my cousins. I am really good at helping family and friends sort out problems.'

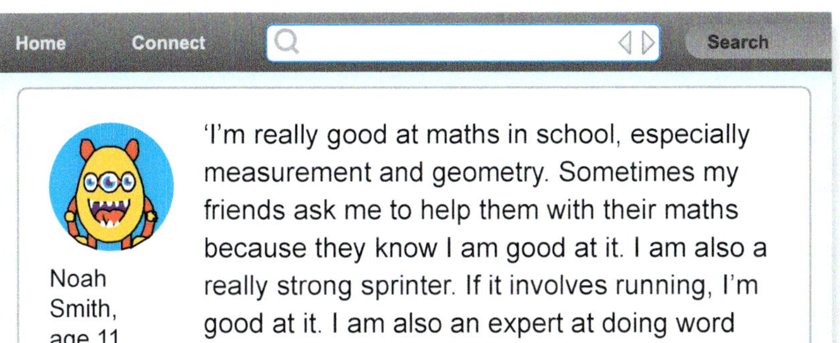

Noah Smith, age 11

'I'm really good at maths in school, especially measurement and geometry. Sometimes my friends ask me to help them with their maths because they know I am good at it. I am also a really strong sprinter. If it involves running, I'm good at it. I am also an expert at doing word searches.'

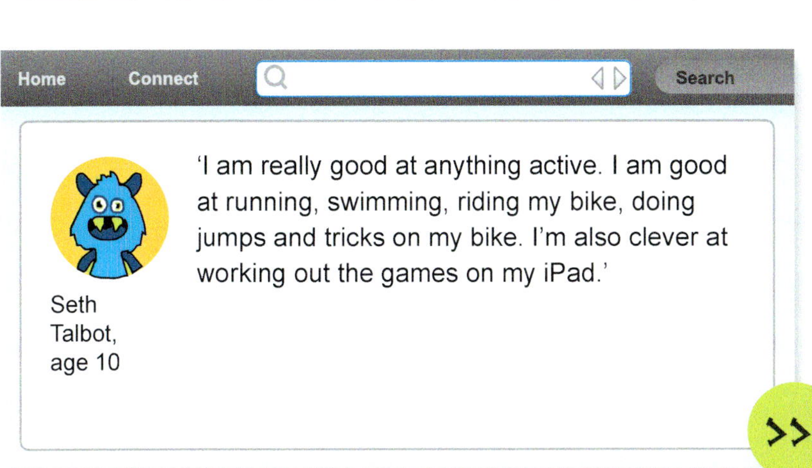

Seth Talbot, age 10

'I am really good at anything active. I am good at running, swimming, riding my bike, doing jumps and tricks on my bike. I'm also clever at working out the games on my iPad.'

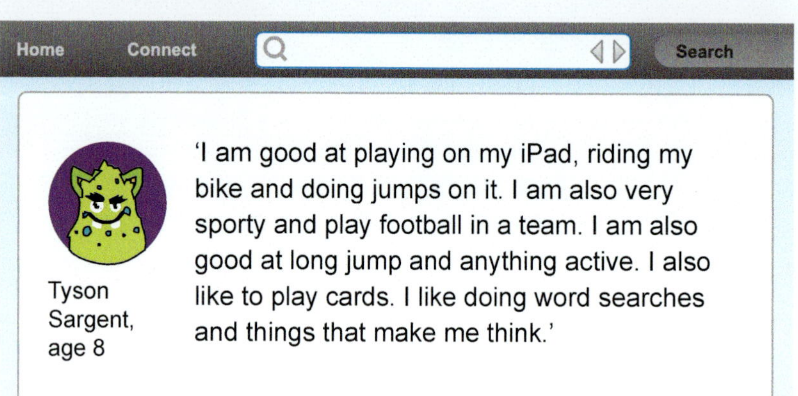

Tyson Sargent, age 8

'I am good at playing on my iPad, riding my bike and doing jumps on it. I am also very sporty and play football in a team. I am also good at long jump and anything active. I also like to play cards. I like doing word searches and things that make me think.'

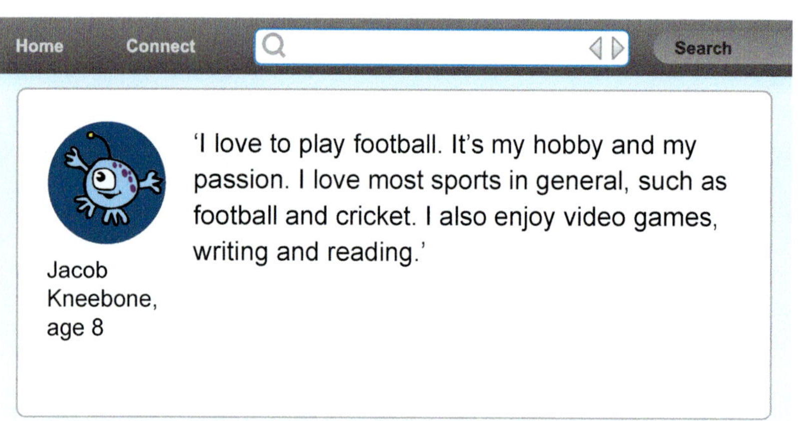

Jacob Kneebone, age 8

'I love to play football. It's my hobby and my passion. I love most sports in general, such as football and cricket. I also enjoy video games, writing and reading.'

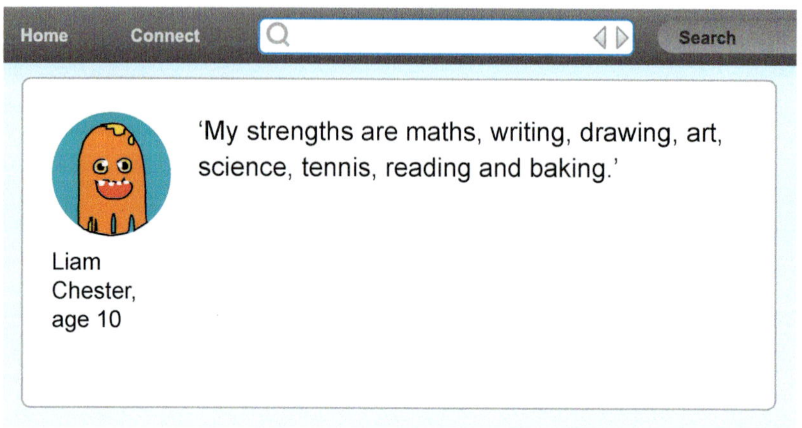

Liam Chester, age 10

'My strengths are maths, writing, drawing, art, science, tennis, reading and baking.'

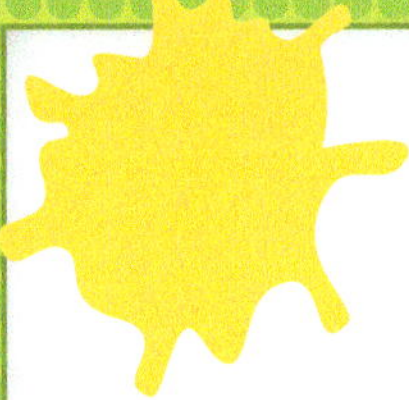

YOU are

YOU are an amazing young man

YOU are one of a kind

There has never been and never will be another YOU

YOU have talents, gifts and dreams that no one else in the world has

YOU were created to make a difference to this world,

even if you don't fully realise it yet

Who YOU are, both on the inside and what you present to others on the outside, matters

YOU are more capable than you think

YOU are stronger than you imagine yourself to be

YOU are kind

YOU are brave

YOU are full of the most amazing potential

YOU are a gift to this world

Just because YOU are in it

Your character

So what is your CHARACTER?

In really simple language, it is who you are and what you stand for. Your character can be described as WHO you are when no one is watching.

Friends and family might describe your character using words such as LOYAL, HUMOROUS, CHEEKY, SMART, SENSIBLE, SENSITIVE, OUTGOING or even QUIET. Think of some characters you might see on television. If you have ever watched the show *The Simpsons*, you will know of Bart. He is a cheeky boy; some would say that he is dishonest, sneaky and rude to his father. He may portray certain characteristics to his dad, Homer, but display other traits to his mum, being generous, loving, and helpful.

For example, someone might act like a loyal and caring mate to someone, but then talk badly about him behind his back or deliberately exclude him from group activities. That behaviour would reveal someone's true character, namely that such a person lacked loyalty and honesty.

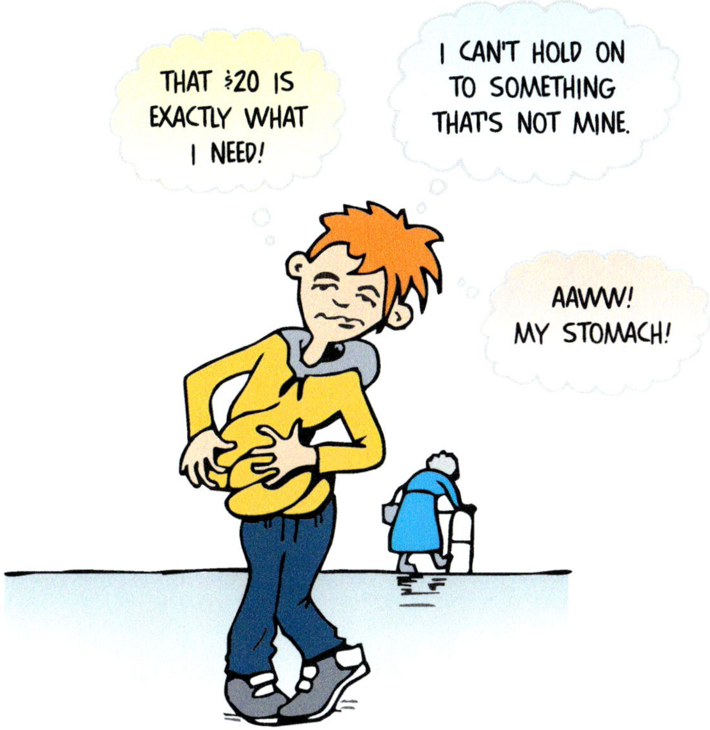

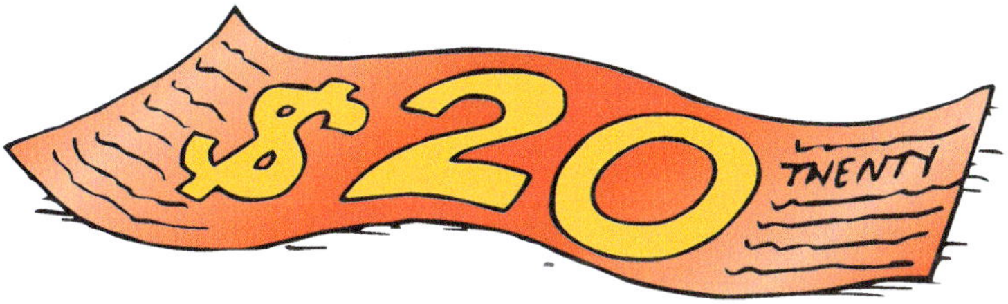

Imagine for a moment that you are walking around the local shopping centre. You notice an elderly lady nearby and see that she drops a twenty-dollar note from her handbag while reaching to get her purse. The money falls on the ground near you, but the woman doesn't notice and continues to walk away.

You have a choice to make.

You can choose to pick up the money and quickly put it in your pocket.

> ***'No one will see me,' you may think to yourself. 'Besides, I've been saving up for a new Playstation game for ages... and that $20 is exactly what I need!'***

It's now that CHARACTER kicks in.

> ***'I can't do that,' you remind yourself. 'I'm an honest person. That's what people notice about me. I can't hold on to something that's not mine.'***

You make the right decision, and run after the woman.

> ***'Here you go,' you say to the shocked woman when she turns back at the sound of your running feet. 'You dropped this 20-dollar note.'***

It can be hard to make a decision like that, putting your character ahead of some selfish desire. It might even be tempting to lie, hiding the truth to protect your reputation in the face of a challenging situation. But it is the RIGHT THING TO DO, and you will be proud of yourself for putting character first.

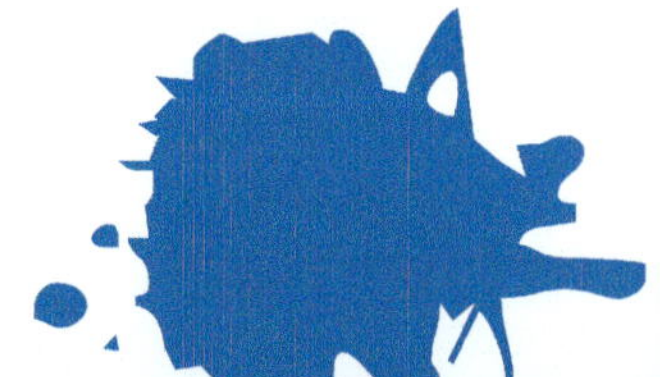

What is your personal brand?

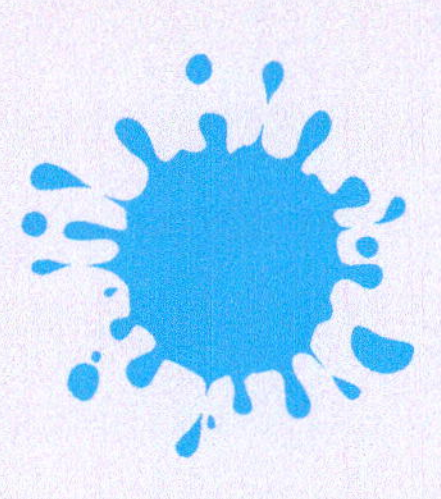

A BRAND is a word, picture or symbol that we instantly recognise as belonging to a specific product or service. For example, most of us — when riding in a car — would know what giant golden arches up ahead would symbolise: McDonald's!

For you, a brand might come in the form of a particular item of clothing because you like the look it represents. Some people, for example, will only purchase a specific brand of television, mobile phone or fridge because they know that this specific brand stands for quality or is built to last.

HEY J!
JULES-MAN!
HEY! J-DOG!
DUDES! IT'S J-MAN!

>>>

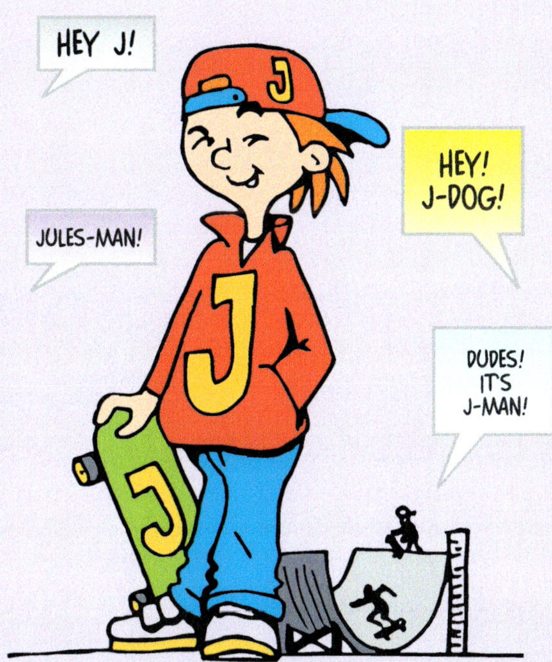

Each of us has a personal brand that we develop from an early age. It is called our REPUTATION. This continues to develop as we grow older. It's what people recognise about us — most often revealed by the words they use to describe us when we are not around.

Think about this for a moment...

If you were to develop a symbol, a group of words or a specific picture to represent YOU and YOUR BRAND, what would it look like? Perhaps it would include three words describing you. It might be in your favourite colour, featuring your favourite sport.

Your brand

On the next page, draw something that represents your brand: WHO YOU ARE. It might include your personal motto — meaning a phrase that describes how you live your life, or what you stand for. Famous company, Nike, merely says on a lot of its marketing material – JUST DO IT – a simple motto of what it represents.

If you were to come up with your personal motto, it might be something like: DO your best with what you have been given.

My personal motto or logo

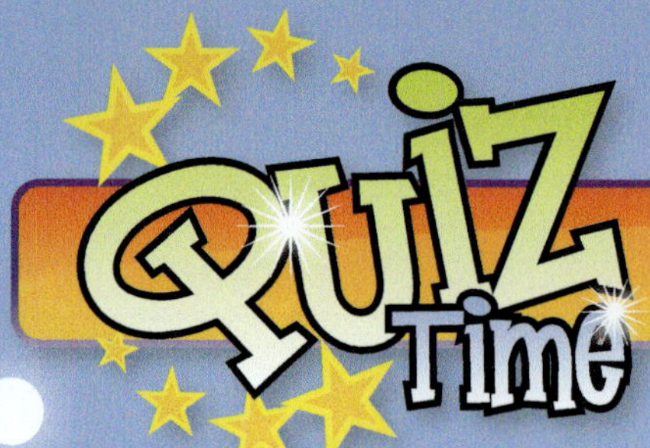

Your character... What would you do?

1) The day the fun ball burst:

You ask Campbell if you can borrow his soccer ball. He only recently received it for his birthday. He is a great mate and of course he agrees to loan it. During recess Sam kicks the ball out of bounds and runs off. You find it and discover that the ball has burst. Your reaction?

A. Tell Campbell that some random guy kicked it into the bush and you assumed it had been returned by the time the bell went.

B. Tell Campbell that it did get kicked out of bounds and that you could help find it together at lunch — even though you've already 'hidden' the burst ball in a bin to avoid confessing the truth.

C. Tell Campbell what happened as soon as you see him. You apologise, but promise that you will replace the soccer ball as soon as possible.

2) The case of the annoyingly neat mother: Mum asks you to clean your room and put all your clothes and books away. What do you do?

A. Go into your room and collect the piles of clothes and books as quickly as you can, shoving them all in your wardrobe (behind boxes so she won't see). You want to get back outside and finish your game.

B. Tell mum that you will, but she has to remind you at least four times throughout the day until you give in and do a quick tidy up.

C. Tell mum that you will do it straight away and spend the next hour cleaning up. You are happy with the result.

3) The one about the teacher who asks for your homework: You arrive at school and realise that you have forgotten to complete your homework. The teacher begins class and asks you where yours is. You...

A. Put on your most relaxed face and tell your teacher that you did the homework, but left it on the kitchen bench at home.

>>>

B. Tell the teacher that your homework must be in your schoolbag, enabling you to go outside and check. Pretend to search through your school bag. Come back in and claim another person must have stolen it.

C. You are honest with your teacher, and tell her that you completely forgot to do it, asking if you can have an extra night to complete the work.

4) When the biscuits go missing:

You arrive home from school and find a packet of chocolate biscuits in the pantry. They look delicious. You are hungry. So, you open the packet and eat three in a hurry. When mum comes home, she is angry when she realises that someone opened the biscuits. She planned to take them to a meeting that night, and asks you directly if you opened them. What do you do?

A. Deny opening them. When mum asks you a second time, deny it again. You are more worried about getting in trouble than lying about it.

B. Tell mum that you saw the opened packet when you arrived home from school. You also add that you're fairly sure your older brother ate the biscuits.

C. Tell mum straight away that it was you who opened and ate the biscuits. Explain that you should have waited and asked her first.

Analysis

* If you answered A or B throughout this quiz, your true character isn't terribly honest. You would rather think through other options than tell the truth straight away.

Try to work on telling the truth first of all. It will make you feel a whole lot better and you will be known as a person of an honest and truthful character.

* If you answered mostly or all Cs, congratulations! You have an honest character and take telling the truth seriously, no matter what the consequences are.

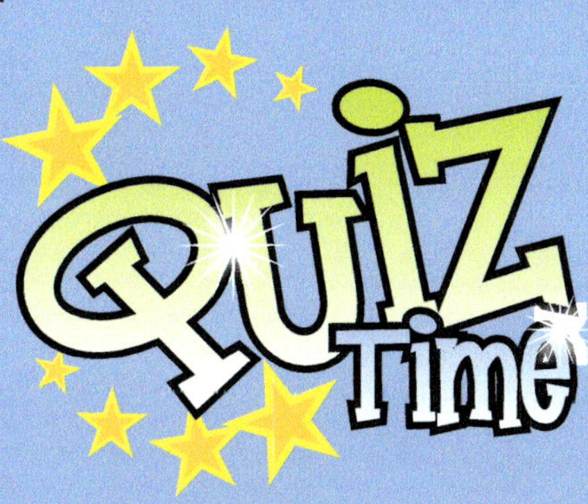

Integrity

My son loves soccer! On a family holiday once, his eyes caught sight of a ball in a shop and he just had to have it.

'Hey Mum,' he said. 'Can I go and buy that ball?
I've got my pocket money with me.'

'Okay,' I said. 'We'll wait out here for you.'

A few minutes later, he emerged with TWO purchases — one was the soccer ball, the other a tasty chocolate bar. My first thought was to speak with him, suggesting he might have thought to buy something for his sister with his loose change and not just think of himself.

'Mum, guess what — ' *(this will be a good one, I thought).* 'The lady in the store was going to charge me $2.95 for the soccer ball. But I remembered that it was actually $3.95 from the sign on the shelf. I told her, too,' my son explained. 'And she was really impressed: "Well, you ARE an honest boy!" she told me. "For that, you can have a chocolate bar as your reward!"'

My son showed integrity and he was rewarded for it.

Integrity is the word that describes your HONESTY and VALUES. It is what defines you as an honest and reliable person, a person whose actions match their words. We all want to be seen by others as people of integrity — it all comes down to what you actually DO, not just what you SAY.

That day, when my son showed integrity, it made me proud to be his mother. I told him that he had proven to himself that he was an honest person, by his WORDS and ACTIONS. It would have been quite easy for him to purchase the ball at the lesser price offered. **Who would have known?**

* * * * * * * * * * *

Imagine you have arrived at school. The moment you get to your seat, you get a sinking feeling: 'Oh no, I watched a movie last night and I've forgotten to do the HOMEWORK for today!'

Now you might be a bit of a legend. You might even be the star student. You can't believe that you let the homework slide this one time.

Then comes the worst thing a teacher can ever utter in such a circumstance: 'Where's your homework?'

Honesty will mean detention.

'Um, oh Miss, I DID do it,' you reply. 'It's sitting on my desk at home, really! I just forgot to bring it in today.'

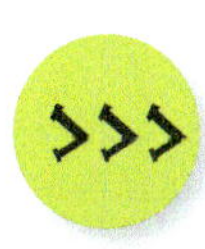

'Miss' looks you in the eye, pauses for a moment and then says you can have an extra day to bring it to school – *'because we all know you are a trustworthy student. Besides, you usually have your homework completed.'*

Now this is an example of your personal integrity at work. Your teacher has come to know you as a RESPONSIBLE and HONEST person. By lying, however, you have put your personal integrity at risk. Your integrity would be much more intact had you told the teacher the truth about not completing your set task. That simple act of honesty, though painful, would have reinforced to your teacher that you are a truthful and trustworthy person.

Classic 'lost' homework reasons...

DOG ATE IT

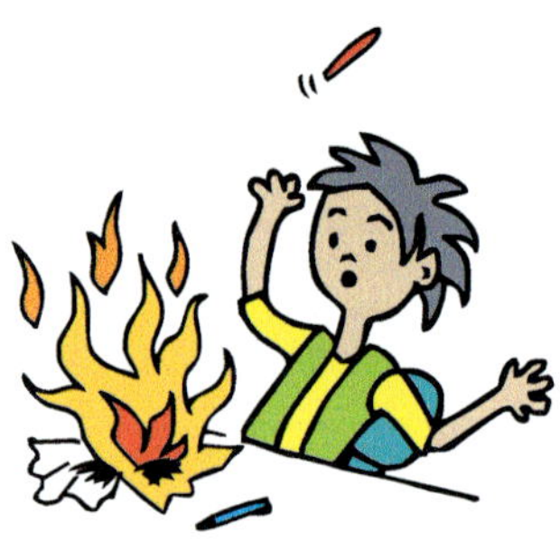

SELF-COMBUSTION

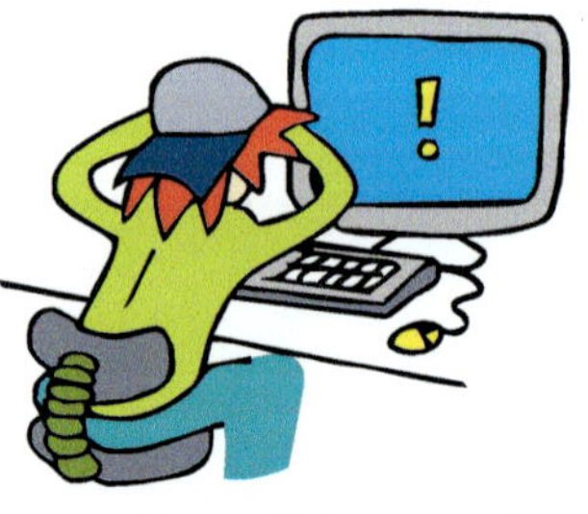

BLUE SCREEN OF DEATH

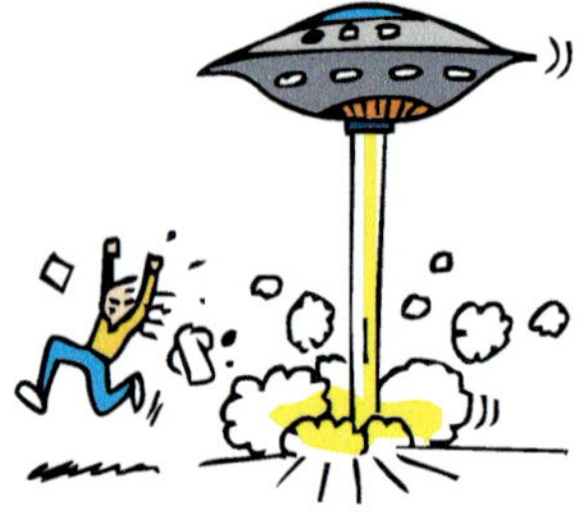

UFO INCIDENT

Accepting consequences

A big part of life and learning comes from accepting the results – or CONSEQUENCES – of our actions and behaviours. So big, in fact, that it happens over many years.

Consequences help us understand what our decisions will lead to. Seeing the effect of a choice helps us to learn what happens when we do something, or when we don't.

For example, if you choose NOT to put your dirty footy uniform in the dirty washing basket, I doubt it will get there magically by itself! One day, when you really need it, that same uniform will probably be just where you left it, in a crumpled mess in the corner of the bathroom – not washed, as you expected.

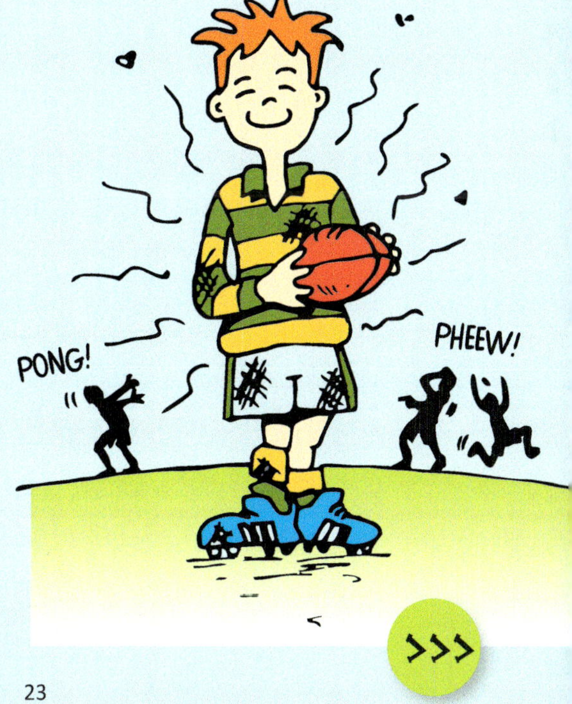

Or perhaps you were too busy watching your favourite television show, and kept putting off completing your maths homework. As a result, you were too tired to finish the homework and went to bed instead. You then have to accept the CONSEQUENCES the next day at school, when you tell your teacher that you didn't complete what was required.

Sometimes, the consequences for our actions, or inactions, can be quite minor. Other times, it can be more serious.

If you are in a hurry to get somewhere, for example, and forget to watch where you are going when crossing the road, you could be hit by a car! That could have disastrous consequences! Or forgetting to put your hat and sunscreen on before enjoying a visit to the beach could mean that you end up being badly sunburnt and in a lot of pain later that evening.

When you need to make an important decision, or even a small one, make sure you take a few minutes to think through what the consequences could be. If you don't like the possible results, perhaps you need to make ANOTHER CHOICE.

Learning valuable life lessons

Jacob and Jesse are great mates and also happen to be cousins. One day, they were both attending a suburban footy match in a suburb which they were unfamiliar with. While there, they wandered into a grassy area away from the game. They noticed one of the home club's footballs sitting half covered in the grass. Clearly labelled with the team's name, they both knew which club owned it.

Jacob suggested they take the football as their own. After all, WHO WOULD KNOW? And surely the club had dozens of footballs already, he reassured Jesse.

Jesse wasn't so sure. He felt like it would be STEALING, even if the club thought that ball was long gone and would never know that these two boys had found and kept it.

Jacob took the ball anyway and hid it under his coat as the boys returned to the car and travelled home.

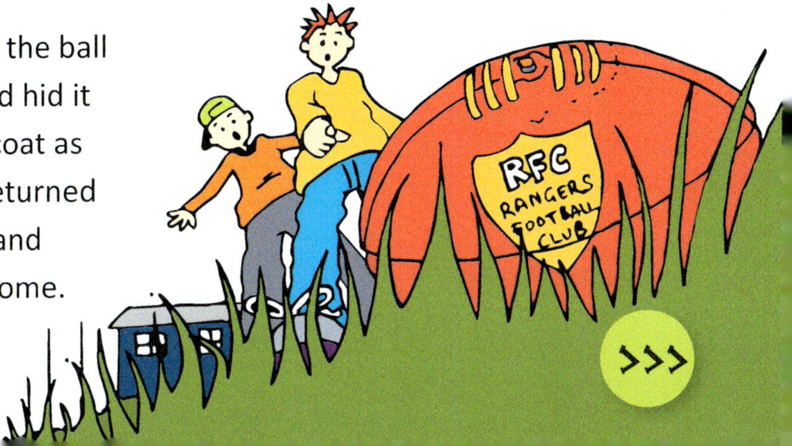

Once back at Jesse's house, Jacob gave the ball to his cousin for safekeeping and it was left in his bedroom.

Two days later, the football that was sitting under Jesse's bed was like a ticking bomb. Just the idea of having a stolen ball in his bedroom made Jesse's stomach feel as if it was tied up in a thousand knots. He tried to sleep for the next couple of nights but it felt like the football was burning a hole right through his bedroom floor. Finally, he woke early one morning and knew what he had to do.

He woke his mum and asked if he could chat with her about something important. Jesse had known that he could talk to his parents about ANY troubles he had, and that there would ALWAYS be a way that difficulties could be sorted out, together.

The problem was, Jesse just couldn't see how this problem could be fixed. He and Jacob had, he believed, done something really wrong. How could the guilt possibly go away?

Jesse sat with tears in his eyes, and explained what had happened that day with his cousin at the footy oval. His mum hugged him and thanked him for being honest about it and coming to her with the problem.

Most importantly, she had the SOLUTION!

She told Jesse that, although the club probably assumed that the football was long gone, it really wasn't okay that they keep the ball. Of course, Jesse already knew this by the way his stomach FELT about his decision.

So his mum explained that it wouldn't be difficult at all to make sure that the football was returned to its rightful owners.

That same day, they looked up the club's address and put the football in a postbox, mailing it back to its owner. Jesse instantly felt much better and knew that he had made the right choice in coming to his mum for advice.

The football was safely returned (probably to a VERY surprised club member who opened the package) and Jesse learned a valuable lesson. Listen to your conscience — that sense of something being right or wrong.

If it doesn't feel right, it most likely isn't.

Jesse also learnt an important lesson about accepting consequences for his actions. Even though he knew deep down that he probably shouldn't keep the ball, he learnt that HE was responsible for the actions of that day and that only HE could take the steps to make it right again.

Stories from boys when they learnt a valuable lesson

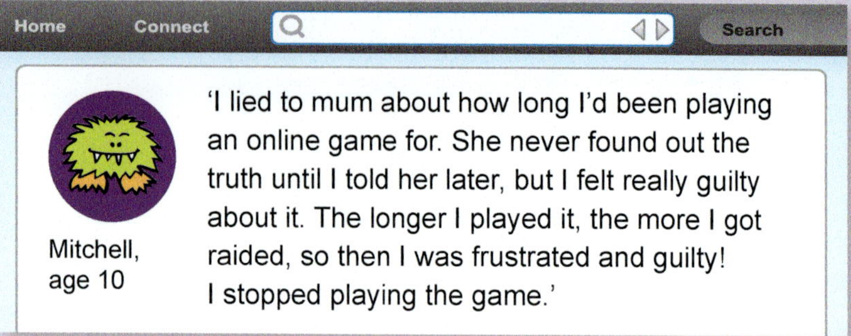

Mitchell, age 10

'I lied to mum about how long I'd been playing an online game for. She never found out the truth until I told her later, but I felt really guilty about it. The longer I played it, the more I got raided, so then I was frustrated and guilty! I stopped playing the game.'

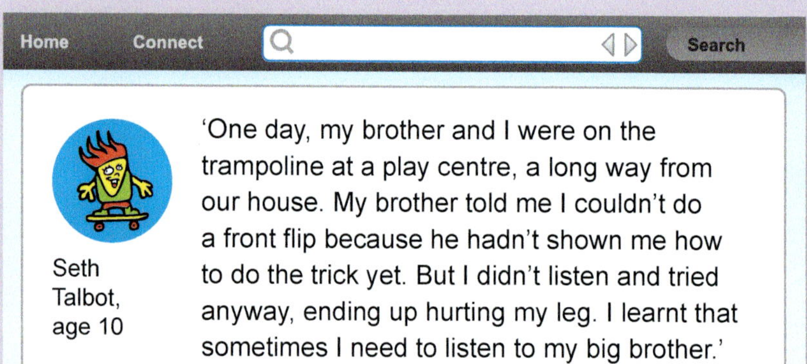

Seth Talbot, age 10

'One day, my brother and I were on the trampoline at a play centre, a long way from our house. My brother told me I couldn't do a front flip because he hadn't shown me how to do the trick yet. But I didn't listen and tried anyway, ending up hurting my leg. I learnt that sometimes I need to listen to my big brother.'

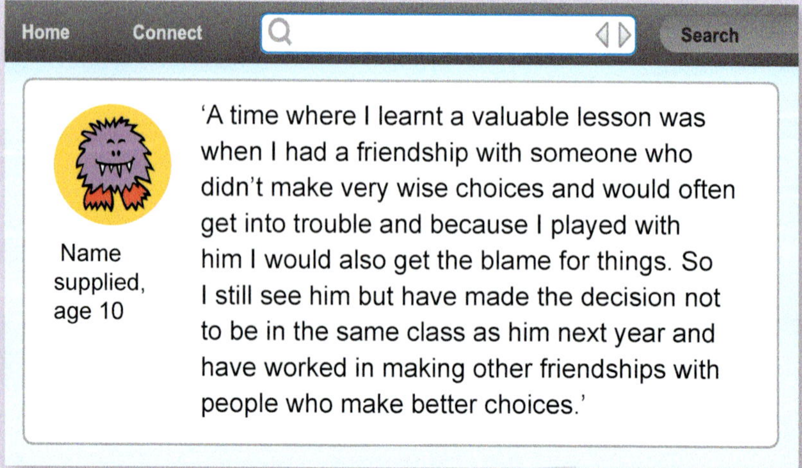

Name supplied, age 10

'A time where I learnt a valuable lesson was when I had a friendship with someone who didn't make very wise choices and would often get into trouble and because I played with him I would also get the blame for things. So I still see him but have made the decision not to be in the same class as him next year and have worked in making other friendships with people who make better choices.'

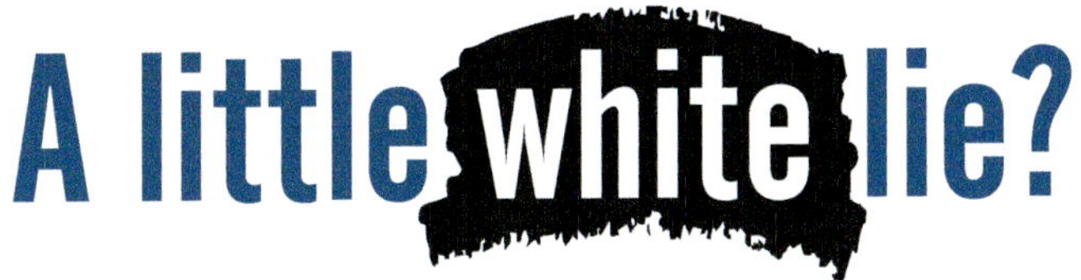

A little white lie?

Have you ever lied?

Well, if you are a human, it is highly likely that you have told at least one – if not MANY – lies in your life so far.

Telling a lie means being UNTRUTHFUL, DISHONEST or BENDING THE TRUTH. The term 'bending the truth' means you aren't lying completely, but explaining away a problem or issue by NOT telling the whole truth, or not giving the FULL explanation.

You may have heard of the term, *'it's only a little white lie.'* This phrase is used when someone wants to justify or make oneself feel better for not telling the whole truth. It can be done to protect someone's feelings.

Think again of that example I mentioned earlier about cleaning up in your room. Perhaps your mum asked if you put all of your clean clothes neatly away in your room. You may have simply gone in there and thrown them all into the bottom drawer in one giant, crumpled mess. That was because you were in a huge hurry to get outside and play.

>>>

You responded to your mum by saying that you had put the clothes away.

Technically speaking, you HAD put them away – somewhere hidden and still messy – but you did not do what your mum asked you to do.

This can still be seen as lying – not telling the FULL truth, or BENDING the real truth – so that it seemed okay.

The problem with lying or being dishonest with others is that you then may not remember what it is you lied about. Lies will eventually get you into trouble. In the example above, it will only be a matter of time before your mum comes into your bedroom to put something away and discover the crumpled mess of clothes that you carelessly threw in the drawer. She will know that you were not truthful.

The second problem is – if and when you DO get found out – you will be known as someone who doesn't always tell the truth if it doesn't suit him at the time.

Think about this for a moment. Is that the sort of person you want to be known as: someone who sometimes doesn't tell the TRUTH?

If you know that you have lied about something, it's not the end of the world. You can make the situation better by being truthful with the person you have lied to.

This isn't easy! It feels scary and nerve racking to go to someone and explain to them that you told a lie.

But if the person cares about you, they will accept your apology and hopefully thank you for being HONEST.

CAN I TRUST YOU WHEN YOU SAID YOU'D TIDY YOUR ROOM?
RUN FOR YOUR LIVES!

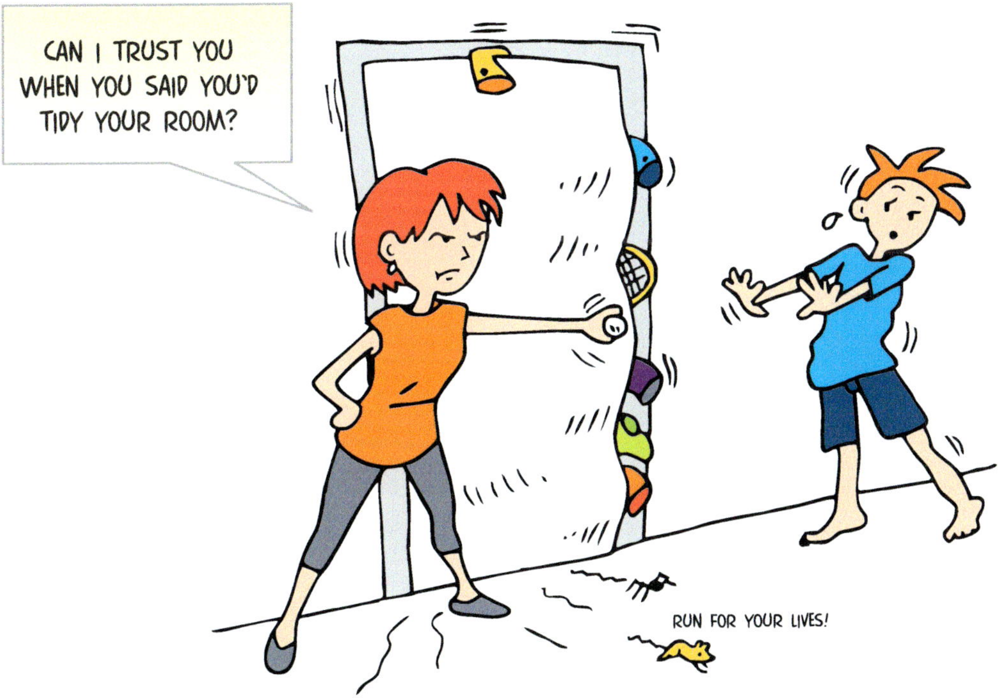

stories about making mistakes and telling the truth

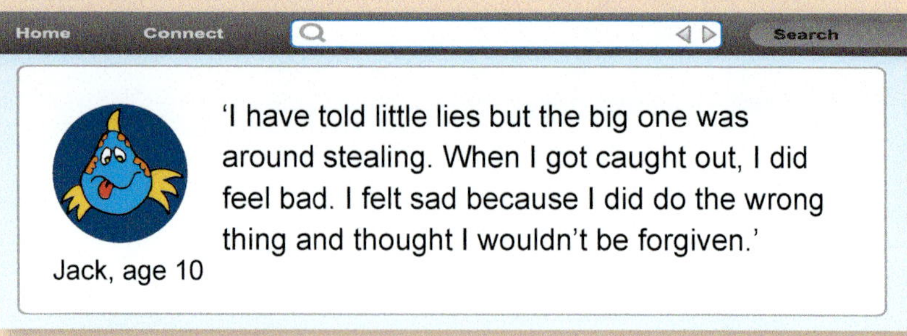

'I have told little lies but the big one was around stealing. When I got caught out, I did feel bad. I felt sad because I did do the wrong thing and thought I wouldn't be forgiven.'

Jack, age 10

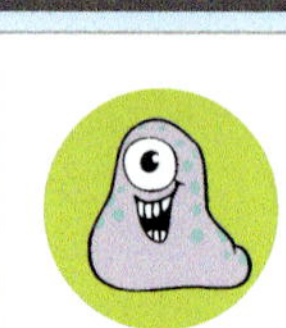

Matthew, age 10

'Once I pushed some big logs off a ledge at school and said I didn't do it. But someone told on me and I had to go to the Principal's office. I learnt not to push things off and also not to lie about what I did.'

Jacob Kneebone, age 8

'Once I chose to hang around with bad company and did something they did. We stole and got caught. Mum and dad made me take the item back and pay for it. I learnt that it wasn't okay to steal, but also it isn't always good to follow friends, knowing what they are doing is wrong. I learnt that I need to set the example.'

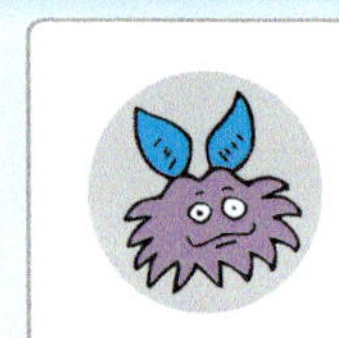

Name supplied, age 7

'I once broke my brother's toy and when mum asked me if it was me, I said "No." Mum then found out and I got into trouble. I try not to lie anymore because mum just always knows. So there's no point in lying because I'll get in trouble.'

Home Connect Search

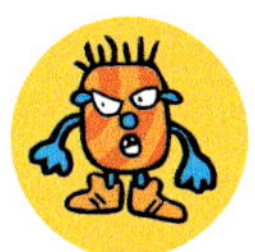

Samuel, age 7

'I once told a lie when mum asked me if I ate my lunch at school. I had already thrown it in the bin. When I told mum the truth, I got in trouble and had to make my own lunch the next day as punishment. I learnt not to throw out my lunch and also, if you lie, you won't have any friends.'

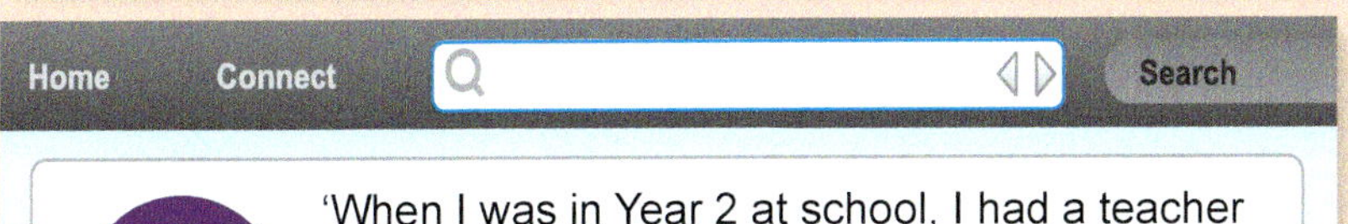

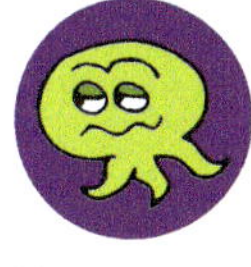

Name supplied, age 12

'When I was in Year 2 at school, I had a teacher for Chinese who would hand-draw stars on my work when I had done well. We would then be rewarded for the amount of stars we had on our work. I soon taught myself to copy her hand-drawn stars and added a few extra. The teacher never found out, but I eventually told my elder brothers one day. They told me off so harshly that I decided it just wasn't worth doing it any more. It just wasn't worth the trouble!'

Home Connect Search

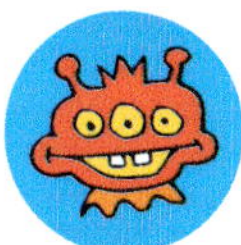

Josiah, age 8

'I stole a Pokemon game card from my mate's collection. My mum found it and asked if I had taken it. I said, "No. Toby gave it to me." My mum said she would give Toby a call and double check. She didn't believe me. She knew it was a card I really wanted. I didn't want her to call him, so I admitted I stole it. She made me give it back the next day with a letter of apology plus two of my favorite Pokemon cards. Mum was very angry that I lied. It made things much worse. I learned my lesson and I haven't stolen anything since.'

Treat others well

It doesn't cost you anything to treat others with RESPECT and KINDNESS. You should always be 'the bigger person' and treat other people as you would like to be treated.

That even means being nice to a replacement teacher coming into your classroom for the day, the person delivering your mail or the opposition player on a sports team. Always treat people respectfully and notice how such kindness and respect returns to you. It's a lot like the old expression, 'What goes around comes around.'

When faced with any kind of connection with someone else, you will always have a CHOICE. You can treat others with respect and kindness, or you can pretend that they do not matter. You can be certain that you will be treated exactly as you treat others.

'"Love your neighbour as yourself." There is no commandment greater than these.'

Mark 12:31 (NIV)

Sometimes, a friend or classmate might not be kind to you. This can hurt your feelings. Does it mean you should treat that person unkindly too? 'At least he'll understand what I felt like,' you may think.

Of course not! If someone treats you badly, that says a lot more about the other person than about you. In fact, most of the time when someone is rude or unkind, it usually means that person has unresolved problems or doesn't feel that great about him or herself.

The best thing we can do in a situation like this is to go ahead and treat the other person with KINDNESS and RESPECT anyway. Yes, it may be hard to do. You may feel angry or hurt that the person was rude to you, but we don't always understand why people treat others poorly.

YOU can control how YOU speak and act towards others.

Always act with kindness and grace towards others, especially those who hurt you because THEY NEED IT MOST!

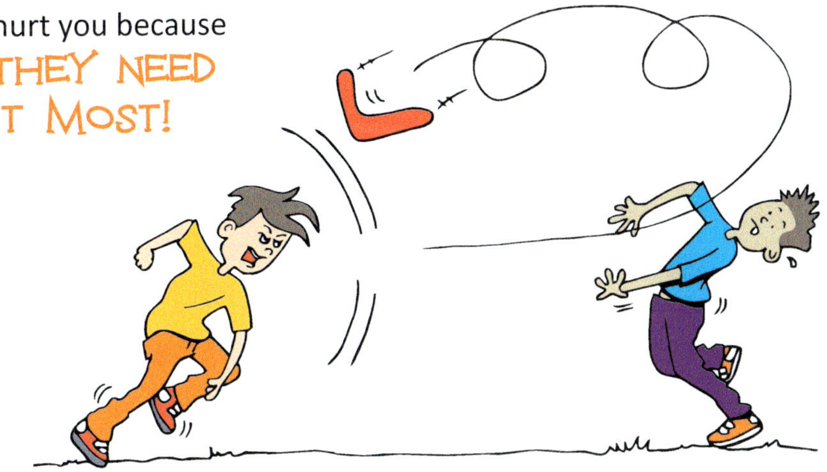

WHAT GOES AROUND COMES AROUND.

Treat others well

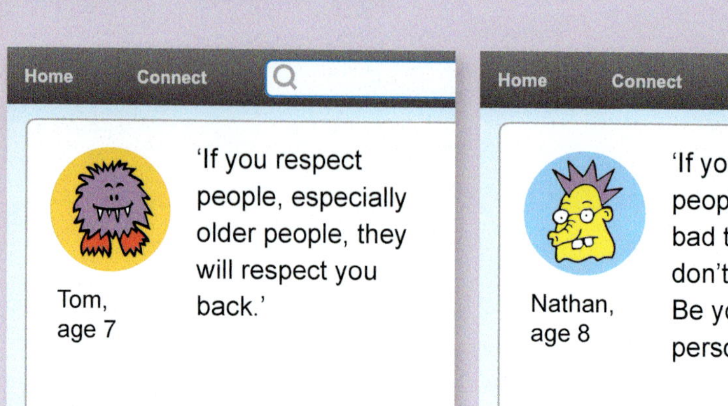

'If you respect people, especially older people, they will respect you back.'

Tom, age 7

'If you see people doing bad things, don't copy them. Be your own person.'

Nathan, age 8

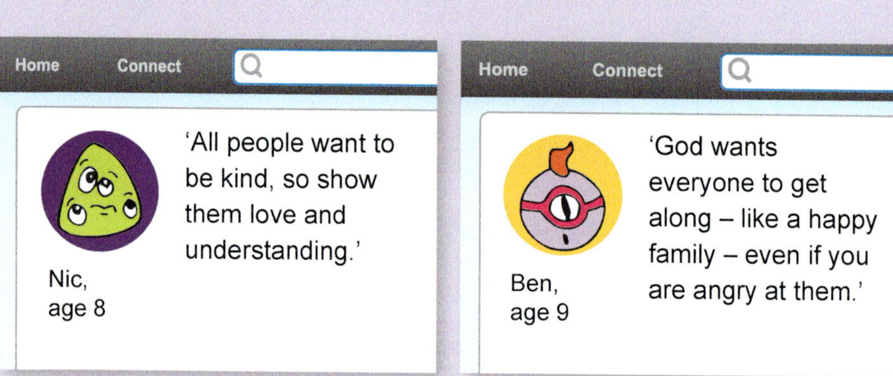

'All people want to be kind, so show them love and understanding.'

Nic, age 8

'God wants everyone to get along – like a happy family – even if you are angry at them.'

Ben, age 9

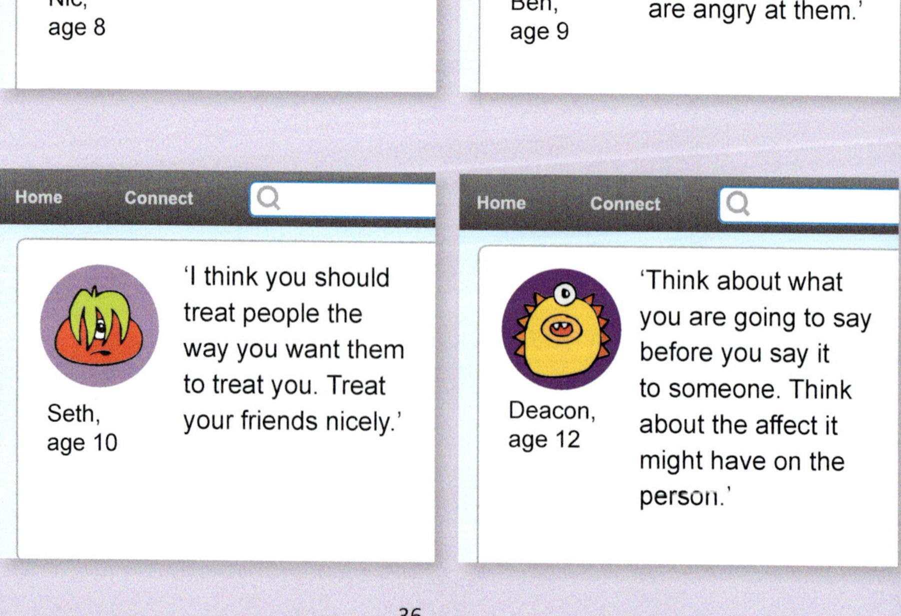

'I think you should treat people the way you want them to treat you. Treat your friends nicely.'

Seth, age 10

'Think about what you are going to say before you say it to someone. Think about the affect it might have on the person.'

Deacon, age 12

Family matters

Family matters

Our family is a very important part of our lives. Families help us to feel LOVED, CONNECTED and a part of something UNIQUE and SPECIAL.

'You don't choose your family. They are God's gift to you, as you are to them.'
Archbishop Desmond Tutu[3]

Your family might be made up of many different people. It may be really small or quite large.

Your family might be made up of your mum, dad, brothers and sisters. It could be your mum, dad and YOU! Perhaps you live with your mum, brothers and sisters, and dad lives somewhere else. You may even live with your dad, or even your grandparents. Maybe you have a guardian, someone who is legally responsible to parent you.

It doesn't matter how your family is made up. It's YOUR FAMILY, whether you all live together in the same house, or different members spend time in other homes.

Some children are lucky enough to be ADOPTED or FOSTERED into a family. They are extremely blessed because they have been brought into something very special and hopefully will feel cared for, loved and supported.

NO, YOU DON'T GET TO PICK 'EM... THIS IS JUST YOUR LOT. ...SIGN HERE.
FRAGILE
THIS SIDE UP
FF
FAMILY FAST

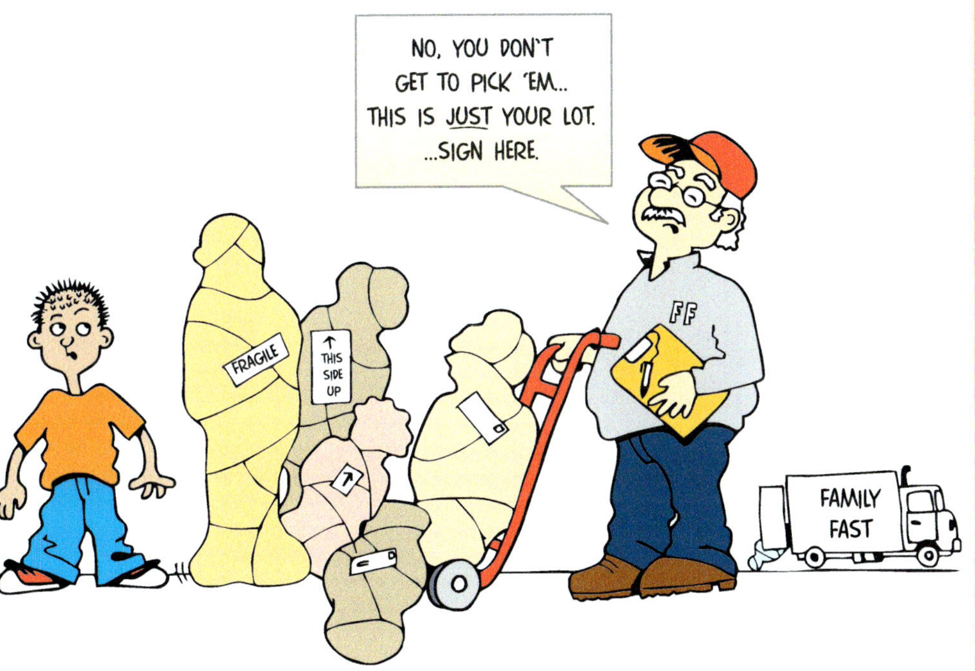

Some people find that the family they become a part of are not even blood-related. This means that they become a part of a family that they aren't necessarily related to, but are just as important nonetheless.

We were never created to live all by ourselves — we need our families to help us get through life, to support us when we have to make important decisions, when we get sick and even when we make poor choices and need a little extra support.

'Family is not an important thing. It's everything.'
Michael J Fox[4]

Being part of a family means you never have to feel totally alone. Quite simply, **YOU BELONG**.

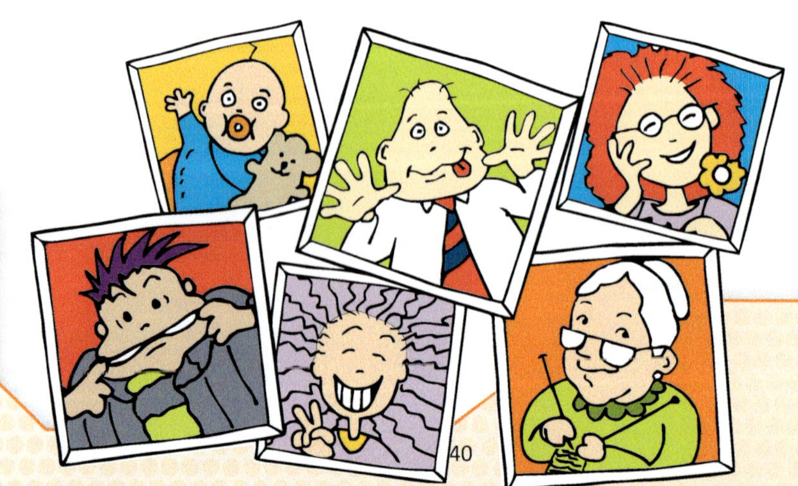

Why my family is so important to ME!

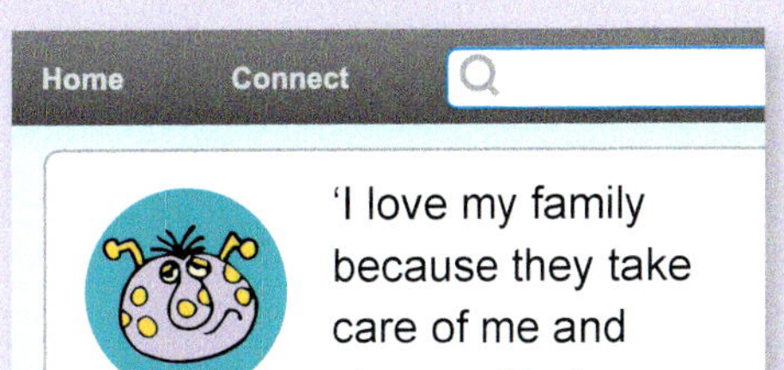

Matthew, age 10

'I love my family because they take care of me and give me big hugs. They help me when I'm hurt or sad. They are there for me all the time.'

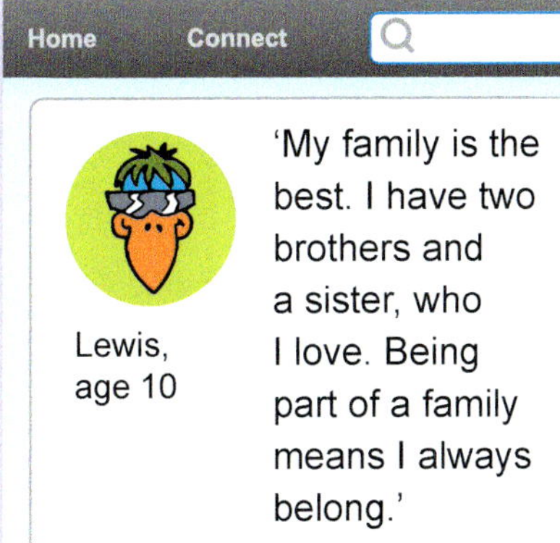

Lewis, age 10

'My family is the best. I have two brothers and a sister, who I love. Being part of a family means I always belong.'

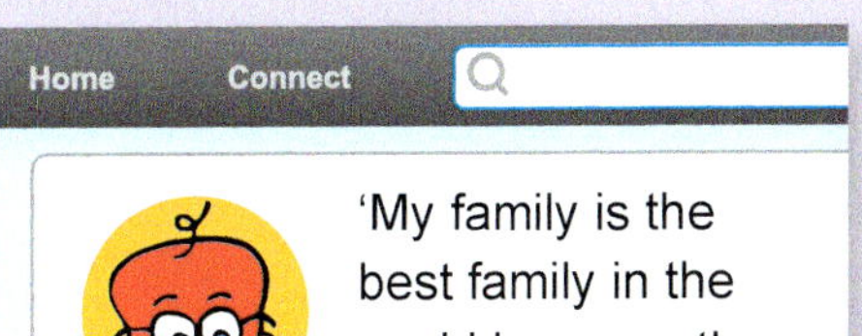

Noah, age 11

'My family is the best family in the world because they are always there for me and always by my side.'

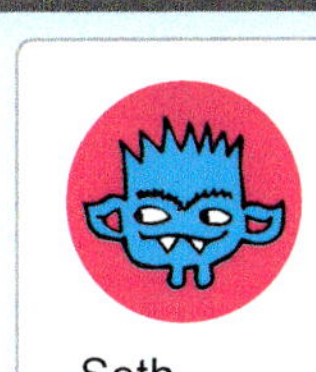

Seth Talbot, age 10

'My family is the best because they care for me and they get me food when I need it. They stand by my side when I'm sick.'

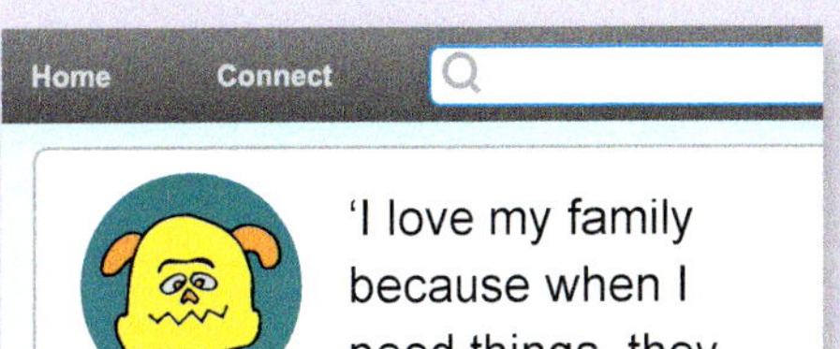

Tyson Sargent, age 8

'I love my family because when I need things, they help me. If I'm hurt, they help me.'

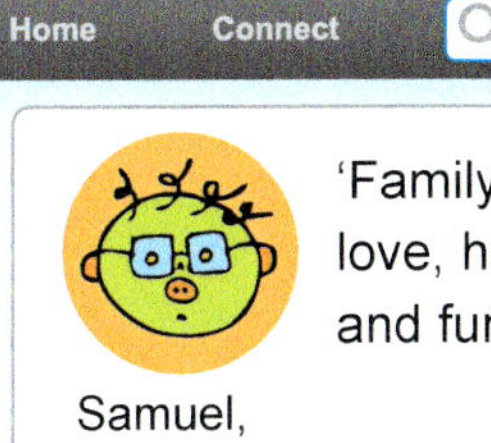

Samuel, age 7

'Family means love, happiness and fun.'

Real WiseGuys

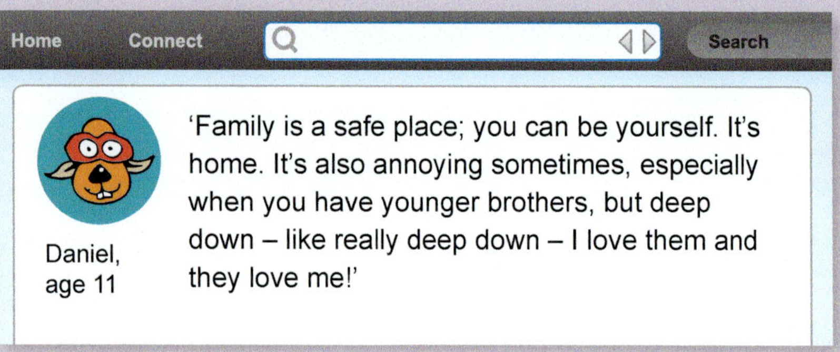

'Family is a safe place; you can be yourself. It's home. It's also annoying sometimes, especially when you have younger brothers, but deep down – like really deep down – I love them and they love me!'

Daniel, age 11

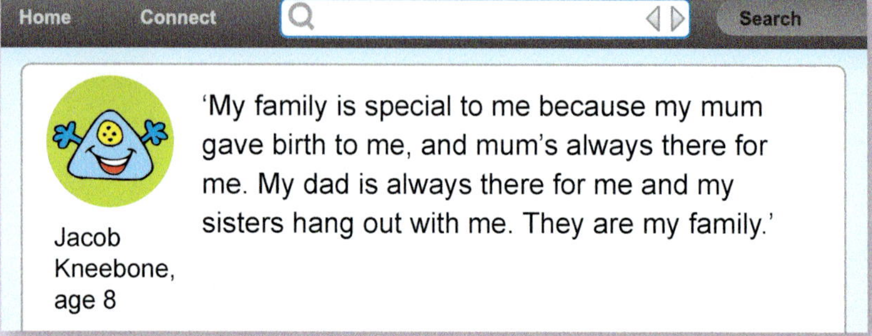

'My family is special to me because my mum gave birth to me, and mum's always there for me. My dad is always there for me and my sisters hang out with me. They are my family.'

Jacob Kneebone, age 8

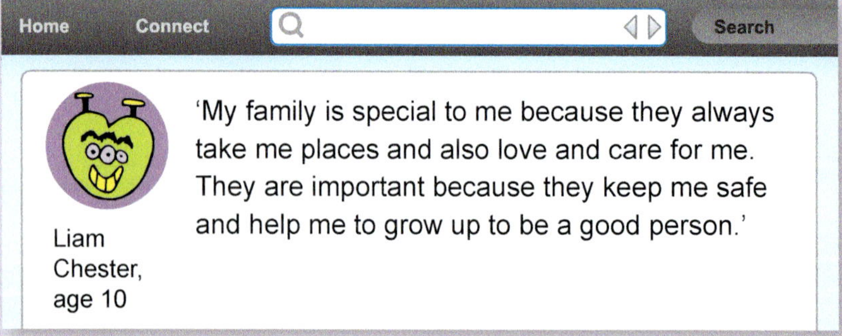

'My family is special to me because they always take me places and also love and care for me. They are important because they keep me safe and help me to grow up to be a good person.'

Liam Chester, age 10

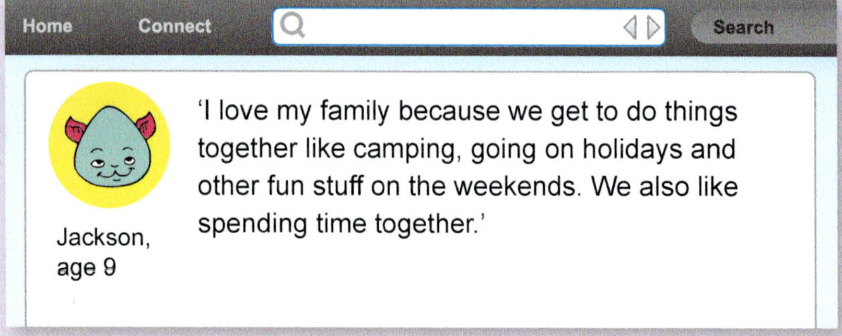

'I love my family because we get to do things together like camping, going on holidays and other fun stuff on the weekends. We also like spending time together.'

Jackson, age 9

Home Connect

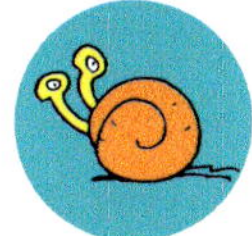

'Family are always there for you, and if they're not, they're not family. They help you and love you.'

Pete,
age 12

Home Connect

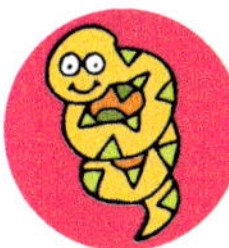

'Family means to me comfort and relationship; someone I feel comfortable with to feel safe.'

Elijah,
age 11

Home Connect

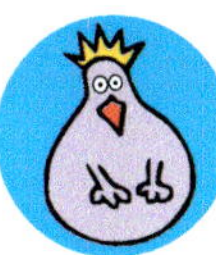

'My family is loving. They watch out for me. They're there for me and are always by my side, even when I don't listen or I am down in the dumps.'

Lewis,
age 9

Home Connect

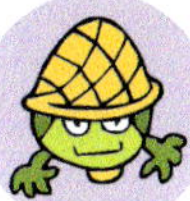

'My family take good care of me. I am the youngest, so I think that's pretty good because I don't have to do as much as my older brothers.'

Liam,
age 7

Home Connect

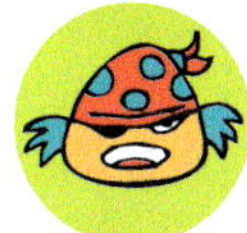

'Family is about spending time together, loving each other and doing things together, like going to new places and seeing new things.'

Xavier,
age 8

Home Connect

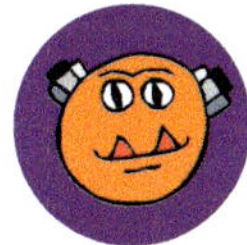

'Family means relatives around me that care about me. I can be confident with them and not shy, and I can trust them.'

Judah,
age 9

Home Connect

'I think family is made up of love, support and guidance; when stuff is good and when things are not so good.'

Mitchell,
age 10

Home Connect

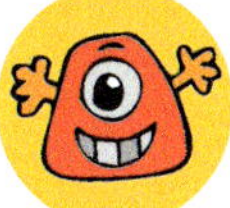

'Family means love. It means being thankful for the people we have in our home, and caring for them, no matter what.'

Isaac,
age 8

Family traditions

TRADITIONS often form an important part of families. They remind us of where our parents and grandparents came from, and help create memories and bonds between each other. They remind us of what makes us WHO WE ARE!

You may have specific traditions created within your family. For example, BIRTHDAYS can generate unique styles and methods of celebration. Maybe you always have a special breakfast together, or you gather in the lounge room early to open cards and presents. Perhaps your mum takes a photo of you standing in your school uniform at the front door before you begin the first day of each school year!

Do you have annual CHRISTMAS TRADITIONS? Do you put the tree up and decorate it in a special way on the 1st of December each year? Do you and your family always attend a Christmas Carols service? Or do you always choose special gifts to give to children in need and deliver them to a charity before Christmas?

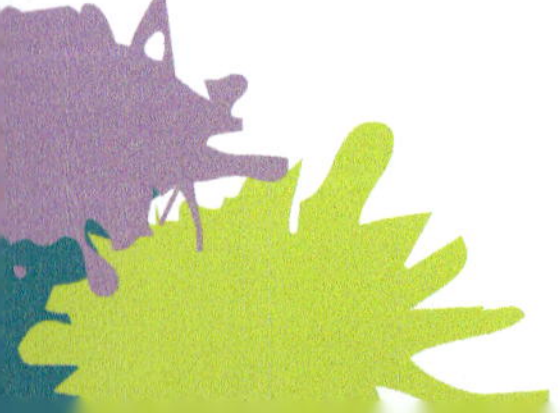

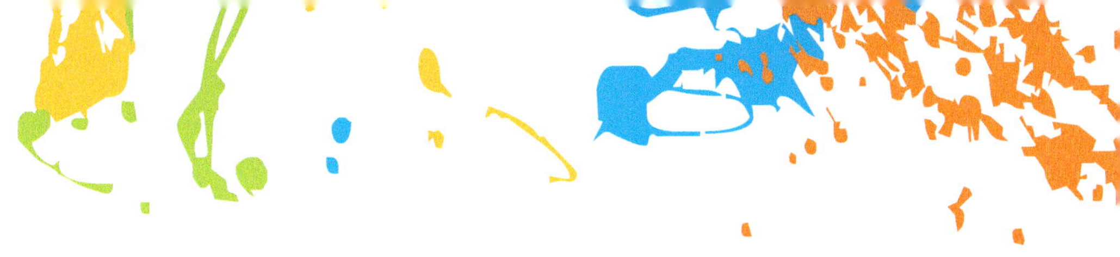

Traditions help reinforce the special unit that is your family. Some families may even observe traditions that have existed for GENERATIONS. Perhaps you even have traditions in your family that began when your grandparents were children.

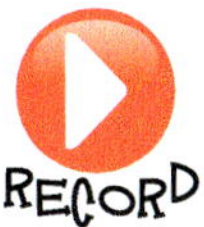

Why not interview your grandparents and ask them what family traditions they had when they were your age? Write the answers below...

stories about family traditions...

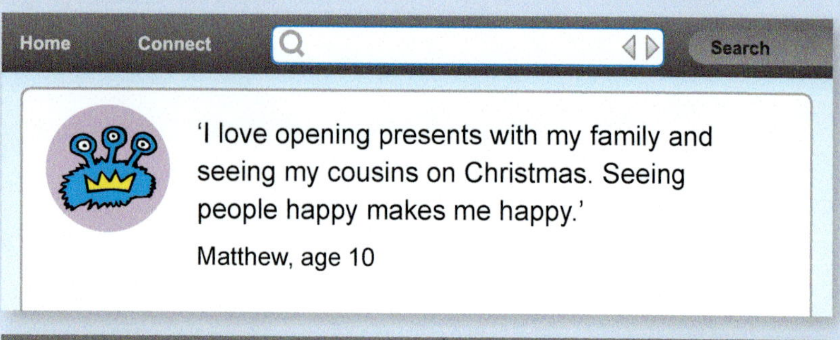

'I love opening presents with my family and seeing my cousins on Christmas. Seeing people happy makes me happy.'

Matthew, age 10

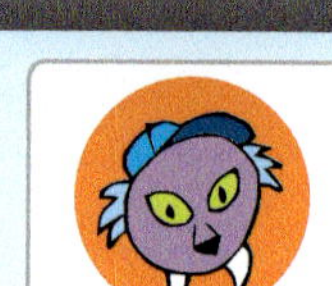

'Every Christmas day, my Nan and Pop come over to visit us at brekky time so we can open presents. They live across the road so it doesn't take long for them to arrive.'

Seth Talbot, age 10

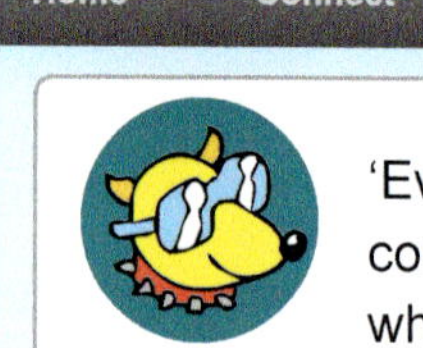

'Every Christmas, we have family members come down from the country and spend the whole day with us. We also always have a real Christmas tree. We go up to the farm near our house and pick it up.'

Noah Smith, age 9

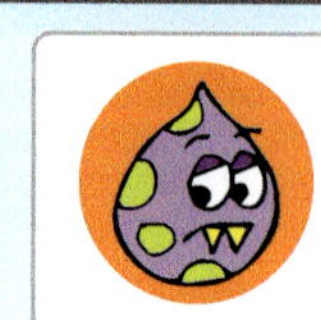

'A tradition in our family is, every Christmas, my Grandma cooks her special Christmas ham. She cooks it beautifully and we get to enjoy it for many days afterwards. It's just not Christmas day without Grandma's ham.'

Jerome, age 9

Home Connect Search

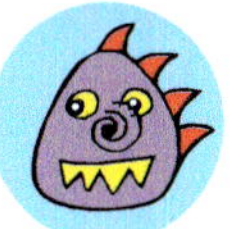

Jacob Kneebone, age 8

'At Christmas time each year, we go away as a family. We also go and look at Christmas lights, set up our Christmas tree together, play board games, watch Christmas movies, have eggnog, visit Myer's window displays and celebrate family. We also donate toys to charity.'

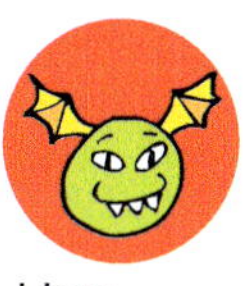

Liam Chester, age 10

'Some of my favourite Christmas traditions are going to my nanna's house and catching up with my cousins on Boxing Day, going to my aunty's house to have Christmas lunch, and going to our church on Christmas Eve to listen to the carols.'

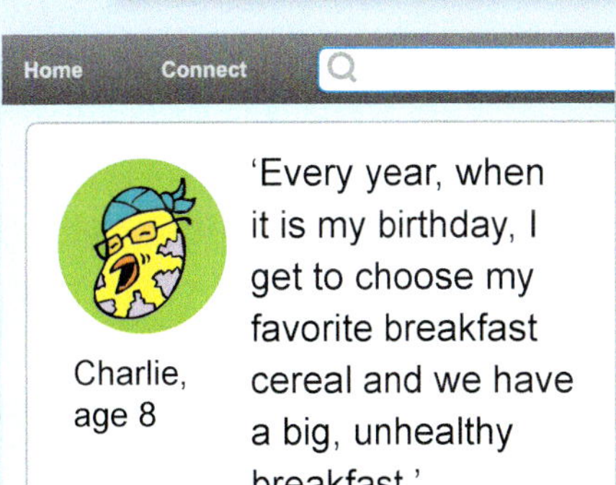

Charlie, age 8

'Every year, when it is my birthday, I get to choose my favorite breakfast cereal and we have a big, unhealthy breakfast.'

Home Connect

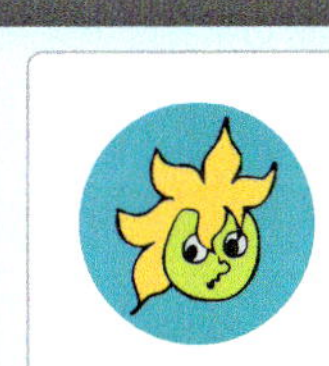

Jake, age 9

'We go to my grandma's house every year on Easter Sunday and we have a giant Easter egg hunt. It lasts for ages because she hides so many little eggs!'

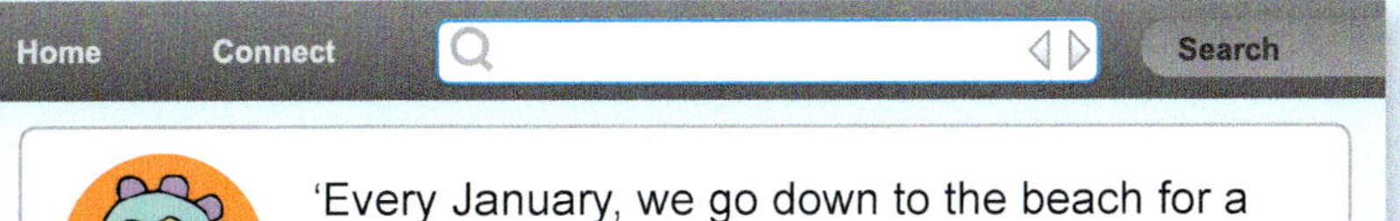

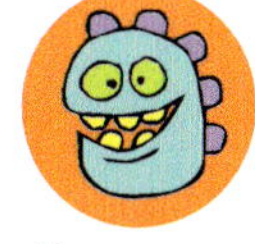

Ben, age 10

'Every January, we go down to the beach for a few weeks to enjoy the summer. We stay in the same caravan park each year and stay up late watching movies together as a family.'

Inspiration about families

'In family life, love is the oil that eases friction, the cement that binds closer together, and the music that brings harmony.'

Friedrich Nietzsche[5]

'Family isn't always blood. It's the people in your life who want you in theirs; the ones who accept you for who you are; the ones who would do anything to see you smile, and who love you no matter what.'

Unknown

'Our family is a circle of strength of love. With every birth and every union, the circle grows.'

Unknown

'The love of a family is life's greatest blessing.'

Unknown

'Family is saying I love you everyday. It is not accepting that your brother or sister is a pain but learning to have fun with them and appreciating differentness. Family is your training ground on how to do life in this world by celebrating the highs and being there for each other in the lows. Family comes first. It is the place you should feel most loved and safe to just be your amazing and talented self.'

Tracey Henderson[6]

'God's favourite fit for each of us is to bring out the best in each other – even if it takes time – and help each other do life through both the happy and sad times. Family is where I can be all of me and be loved for it.'

Shannon Harrison[7]

When family circumstances change

Sometimes, you might find yourself in the middle of a major family change. This can be really, REALLY difficult to deal with.

> 'Do not be anxious about anything, but in every situation, by prayer and petition, with thanksgiving, present your requests to God.'
>
> Philippians 4:6 (NIV)

The family change might be your mum and dad deciding to separate and live apart in two homes. Or perhaps one parent becomes ill, or even has to travel away to work for a lengthy period of time. Maybe a new family member arrives in the form of a baby or foster child. Sometimes, sadly, someone passes away.

There are many ways and situations in which your family circumstances might CHANGE.

Firstly, I want you to know right now that anything that changes in your family is NOT YOUR FAULT! You did not cause it.

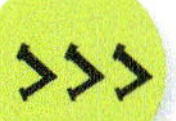

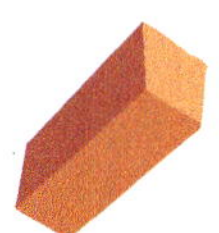

Often, when tough things happen in a family, it is natural to want to blame someone. We can get angry and want to question why it happened. This is perfectly NORMAL.

Sometimes, we might try and BLAME ourselves. But this is not the case. You are just a young boy and nothing you did made this happen. You have to realise that you also cannot change a difficult situation.

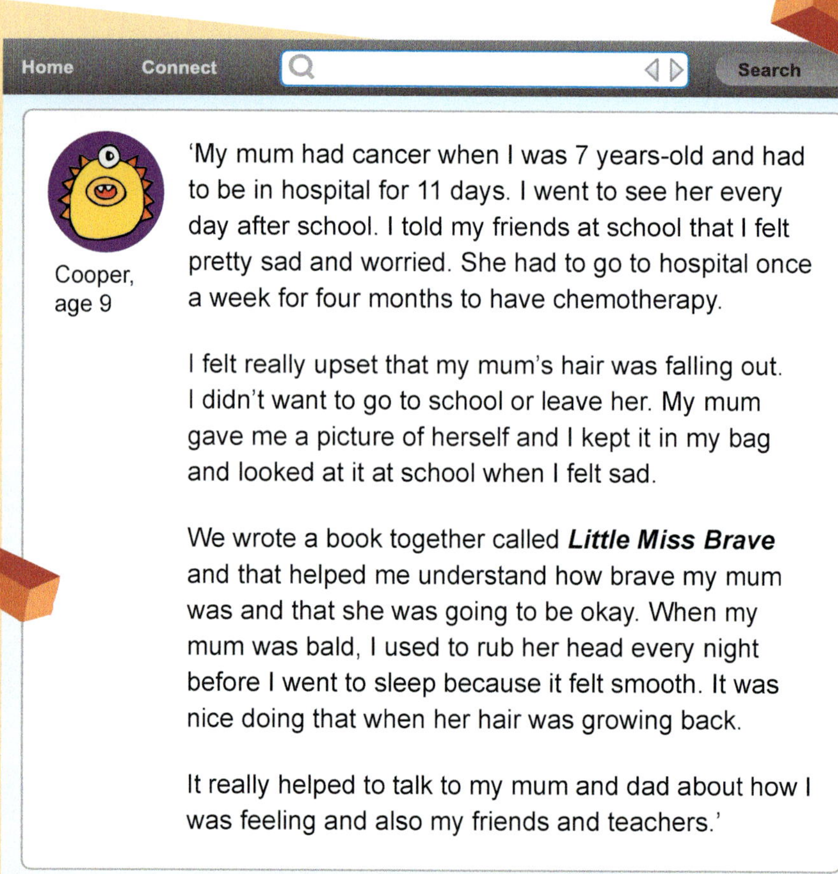

Cooper, age 9

'My mum had cancer when I was 7 years-old and had to be in hospital for 11 days. I went to see her every day after school. I told my friends at school that I felt pretty sad and worried. She had to go to hospital once a week for four months to have chemotherapy.

I felt really upset that my mum's hair was falling out. I didn't want to go to school or leave her. My mum gave me a picture of herself and I kept it in my bag and looked at it at school when I felt sad.

We wrote a book together called ***Little Miss Brave*** and that helped me understand how brave my mum was and that she was going to be okay. When my mum was bald, I used to rub her head every night before I went to sleep because it felt smooth. It was nice doing that when her hair was growing back.

It really helped to talk to my mum and dad about how I was feeling and also my friends and teachers.'

Answers in tough times

What can you do when your family situation changes and you are finding it tough?

- **Surround yourself with positive people** who love you and make you feel secure.
- **Talk:** Find someone who you can talk with about your feelings, fears and how to move forward. This could be your mum, dad, aunt, grandmother, teacher, sports coach, school counsellor or youth leader.
- **Keep doing the things you enjoy:** It's important to keep doing those activities that make you feel happy and keep your mind occupied. Keep playing your sports games. Don't drop out. Hang out with your mates, ride skateboards or bikes.
- **Journal:** Writing how you are feeling is often a great way to get feelings and emotions out. Even if you get an exercise book or notebook, go somewhere quiet and private where you can write your feelings down.
- **Exercise:** Going for a brisk walk or playing sport is a great way to release feel-good chemicals in the brain called 'endorphins'. They can help us keep a clear and positive mindset.
- **Speak positively:** Despite how you might feel about your family, or what you may overhear, try to keep your thoughts positive and speak well about the family members affected.

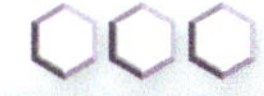

Coping with loss

When a family member or someone special to you passes away

It's a really difficult part of life that sometimes we experience a family member or really close friend passing away. This is a terribly sad fact of life and something that, unfortunately, most of us will experience at different stages of our lives.

'No one ever told me that grief felt so like fear.'

C S Lewis[8]

Sometimes, you may have time to say goodbye, as difficult as this is. At other times, you will have no warning at all. No matter how it happens, it will not be easy. Losing someone we love and care for is HORRIBLE and AWFUL and there is just no way of making this any easier at the time.

When I was younger, my dearest Nan passed away after a short illness. I was able to visit her in hospital in the weeks leading to her passing away, but it still hurt so much when I received news that she had finally gone to Heaven. She had lived a very long and wonderful life, but even still, it was difficult for those of us left behind who were without her.

What can you do to get through the grief?

Firstly, grief – feeling very sad and upset that you have lost a loved one – is a REAL and NORMAL emotion to FEEL. Ultimately, it is healthy to allow yourself to experience such pain rather than hide it.

Yes, it will hurt like crazy, but hopefully soon it will get a little easier to manage. Over more time, it will continue to be less painful. The passing of time will not, however, stop you from MISSING the people who leave. Instead, you will be able to remember the great memories you had with that special person.

'To weep is to make less the depth of grief.'

William Shakespeare (Richard, Henry VI, Part 3, Act 2, Scene 1, line 85)

stories from guys who have lost someone special...

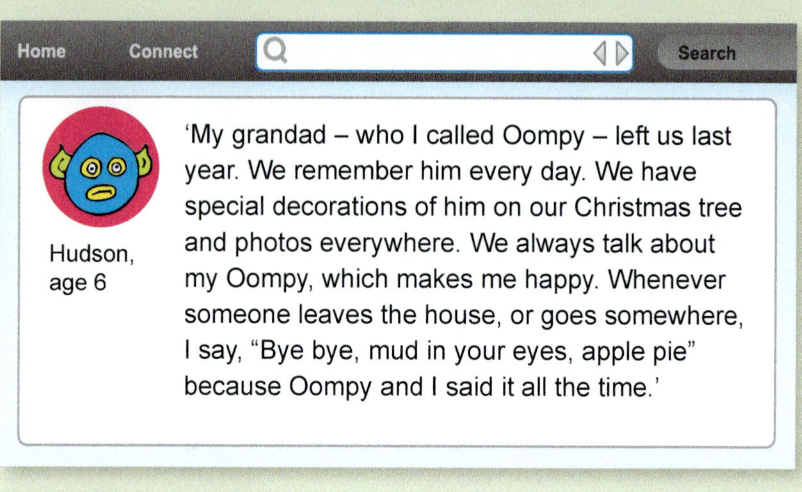

Hudson, age 6

'My grandad – who I called Oompy – left us last year. We remember him every day. We have special decorations of him on our Christmas tree and photos everywhere. We always talk about my Oompy, which makes me happy. Whenever someone leaves the house, or goes somewhere, I say, "Bye bye, mud in your eyes, apple pie" because Oompy and I said it all the time.'

Home Connect Search

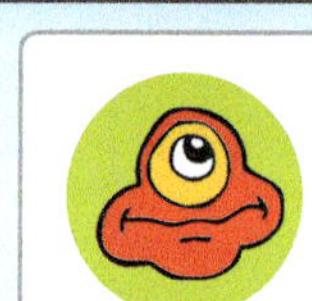

Kai, age 7

'I like my mum to tell me stories about my grandpa, who I miss very much. I like her telling me stories about him, especially stories of him fighting in World War Two.'

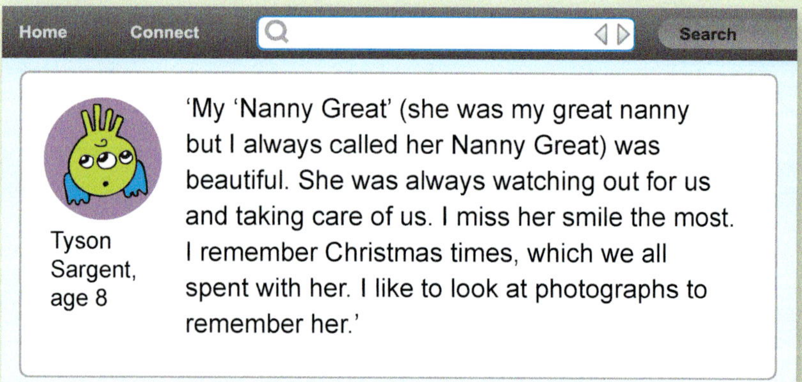

Tyson Sargent, age 8

'My 'Nanny Great' (she was my great nanny but I always called her Nanny Great) was beautiful. She was always watching out for us and taking care of us. I miss her smile the most. I remember Christmas times, which we all spent with her. I like to look at photographs to remember her.'

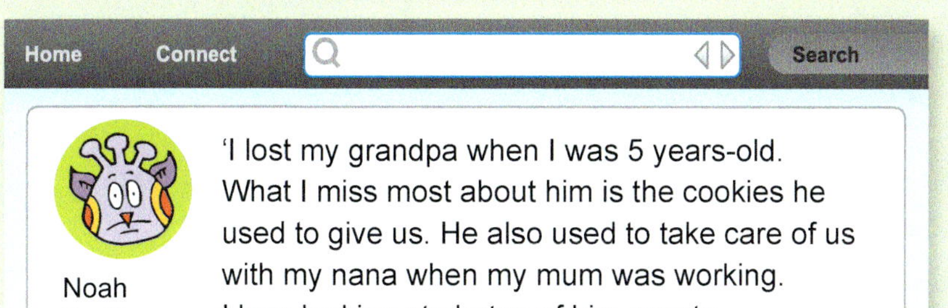

Noah Smith, age 11

'I lost my grandpa when I was 5 years-old. What I miss most about him is the cookies he used to give us. He also used to take care of us with my nana when my mum was working. I love looking at photos of him now to remember him.'

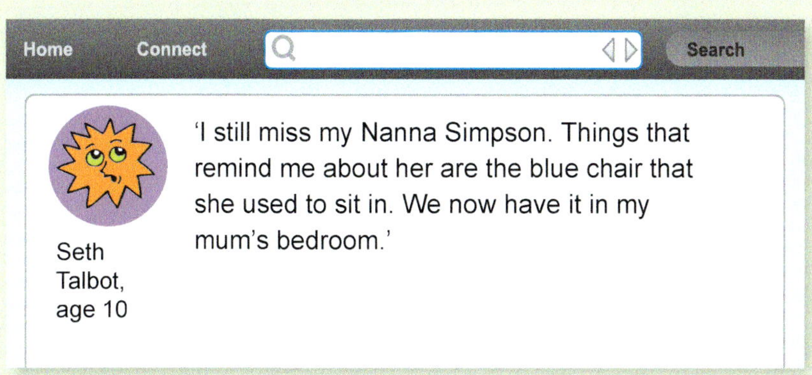

Seth Talbot, age 10

'I still miss my Nanna Simpson. Things that remind me about her are the blue chair that she used to sit in. We now have it in my mum's bedroom.'

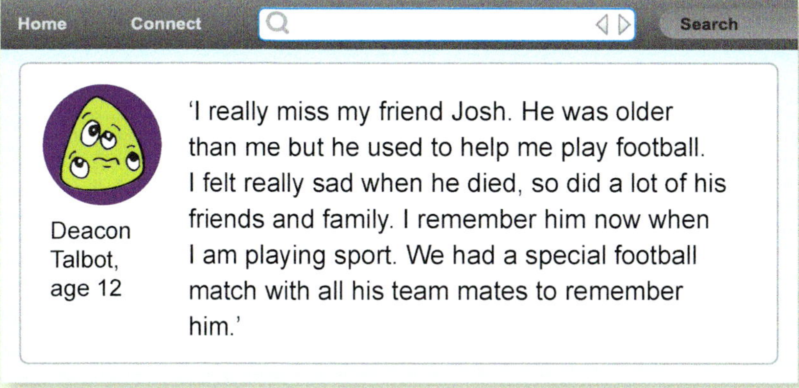

Deacon Talbot, age 12

'I really miss my friend Josh. He was older than me but he used to help me play football. I felt really sad when he died, so did a lot of his friends and family. I remember him now when I am playing sport. We had a special football match with all his team mates to remember him.'

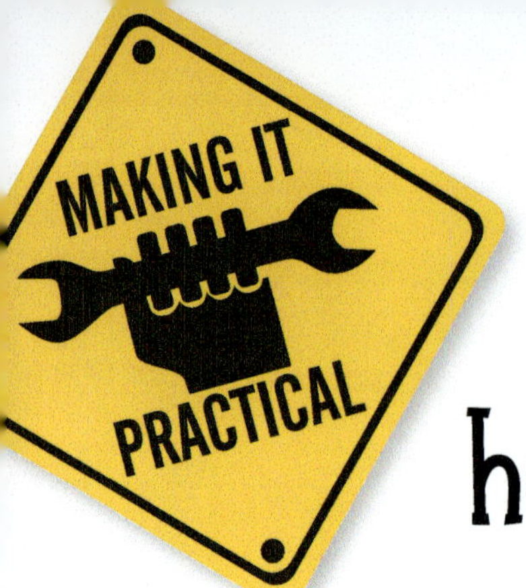

Ideas to help with loss

Plant a SPECIAL TREE or beautiful ROSE in your garden to honour the family member you lost.

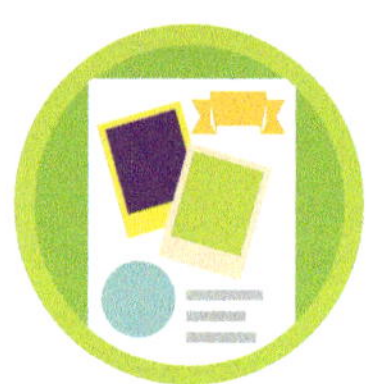

Make a SCRAPBOOK ALBUM of your best and most treasured memories.

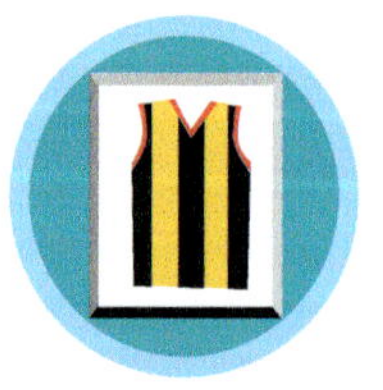

Frame your favourite PHOTO of someone you have lost. Or, if the person loved a sport or team, frame a club footy jumper or cricket top: something to remind you of how SPECIAL that person was. Just seeing the jumper will remind you of the person you miss, remembering how he cheered when his footy team won a game, or funny things that he said when the club lost.

Write your loved one a LETTER, telling that person of your love and what you miss the most. You can keep it close to your heart or put it in a special place.

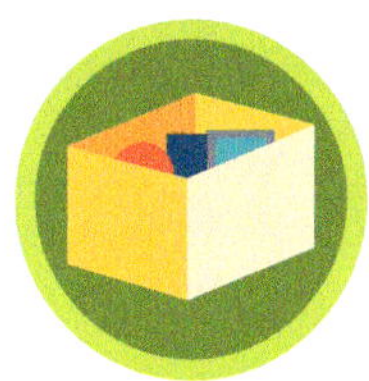

Make a KEEPSAKE BOX. Get a special box that you can fill with precious memories of your family member. Then, when you have a particularly sad day grieving, you could spend time quietly going through your memory box.

PRAY for your sense of loss and for those around you who are also missing that person. Pray for peace that passes understanding over your mind and soul as you grieve.

TALK with others about your missed loved one. Share funny stories and happy memories you shared with that person to keep the memories alive. Talking about the person shouldn't be something you avoid. It helps keep others' memories alive when you share the happy moments that you have.

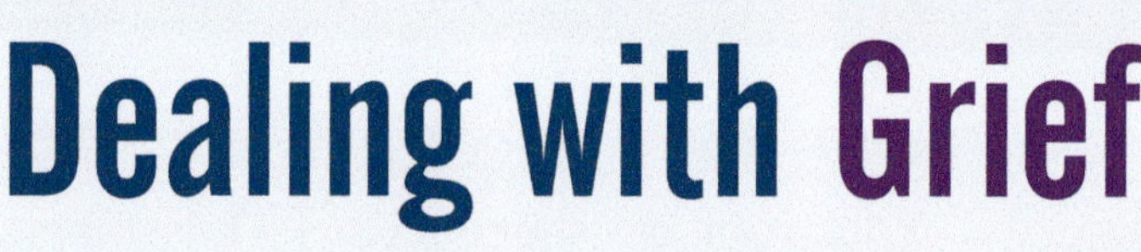

Dealing with Grief

When I was 20 years-old, my best friend in the world passed away. It was very sudden and I thought my entire world had fallen apart. It was really, REALLY difficult to cope with the grief some days.

I remember sitting in my bedroom crying as I listened to songs we had shared and enjoyed together. Thoughts would flood back as tears made their way down my cheeks. Though very sad, just remembering him made it somehow easier over time.

I often felt very ALONE.

Grief is such a personal thing and it's important to know that different people grieve and feel sadness in different ways, and there is NO right or wrong way to grieve for a person who has died.

One thing I did learn was that it was okay to talk about him, as often as I wanted to. I also found it helpful to spend time with his family after he had passed away, because I could talk about him. We could share memories of fun and eventful times together. And it was okay to laugh too! Some of my memories of him were really funny and it was quite okay and good to share these.

Every year, on the anniversary of his death, I always buy a bunch of flowers for his mum and dad and visit them. It is so important to them that his friends REMEMBER him. I am not making it harder for them. They are already feeling sad, but I am actually saying, 'Hey, I remember my best friend and I miss him too.'

Sadness is a normal part of the grieving process. People around you will understand when they see you upset. But if you find that your thoughts are getting sadder, and harder to deal with, it is VERY IMPORTANT that you speak with a friend or trusted adult straight away. This is not something you EVER have to deal with by yourself. You won't be bringing others down with you, I promise. Friends and family would much rather get alongside and support you, cry with you or do things to support you, than know that you have been suffering alone. Please tell someone if you are struggling.

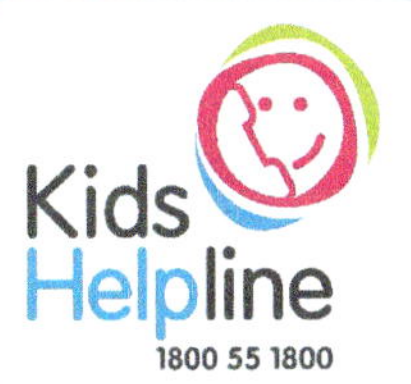

You can also call LIFELINE at any time, day or night. This is a FREE CALL and the people who answer the phones won't try and ring you back or trace the call. They are there to talk with you. Perhaps they will be able to give you some advice to get through the next few hours, days and weeks.

Kids Helpline 1800 55 1800
www.kidshelp.com.au

Taking care of yourself during loss

Being happy or having fun doesn't mean you don't still miss them.

If mates ask you to hang out with them or play a game, don't feel you have to say no, just because you are sad about the person you have lost.

Actually, getting out and taking some time to have fun and enjoy life is the best thing you can do right now. It doesn't mean you have forgotten your loved one, or that you have moved on. It just means that you are giving yourself permission to care for YOURSELF, also. And that is a healthy thing to do.

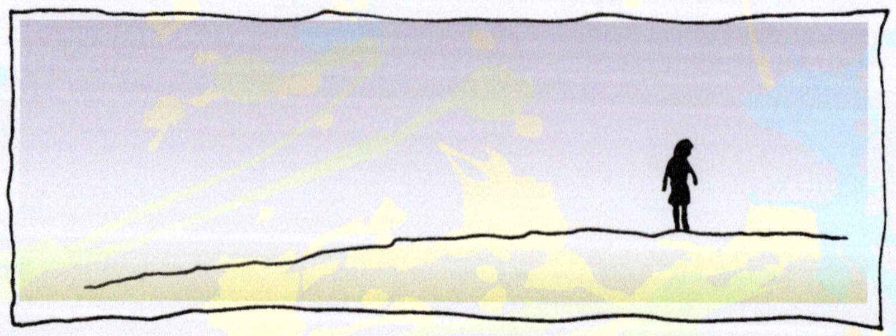

Losing a pet

Losing a pet – whether through passing away or becoming lost – can be **DEVASTATING**. It is literally like losing a member of your family. Our pets form deep bonds and connections with us and it is really difficult to deal with when we have to say goodbye.

We have a beautiful dog, named Ella. She is absolutely beautiful, and because she was born as the runt of the litter, she is forever going to be the size of a puppy. She is definitely an important member of our family. When she wakes each morning, Ella comes and finds my daughter, wherever she is in the house. (She is actually my daughter's pet, but we all share her.)

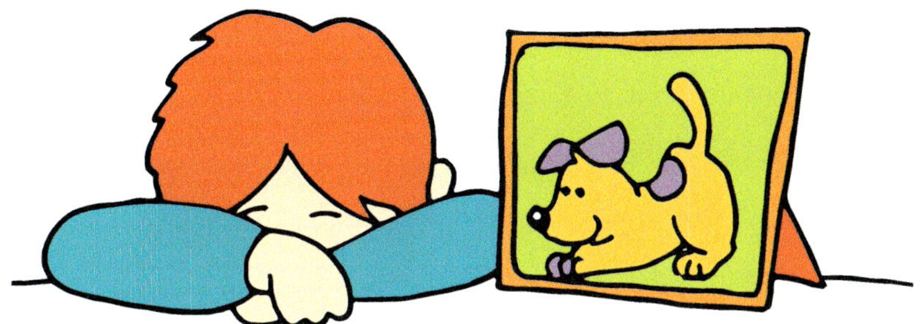

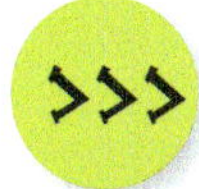

When you are feeling sick or a bit down in the dumps, it's as if she knows that you need an extra measure of affection that day. She will curl up beside you and sleep, just 'being' there for you.

You may have any type of pet: a puppy, a rabbit, even a snake! No matter what type of pet it is, you will still feel a sense of loss and grief when you have to say GOODBYE.

It can be a difficult process to mourn the loss of a pet. Be kind to yourself. It will take time. You can hold on to some cherished memories of your precious pet. The following are a few ideas that you can put into action to work through your loss.

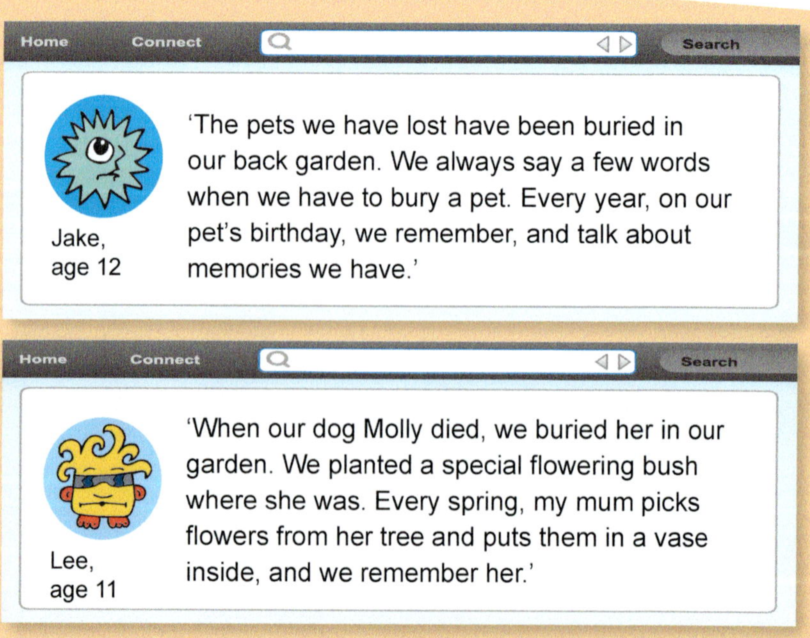

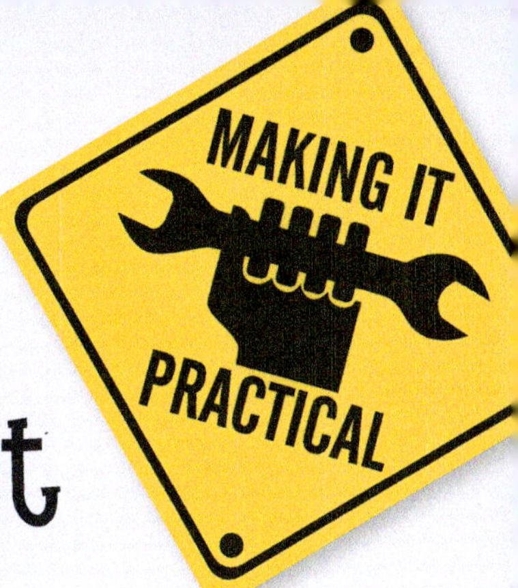

Remembering your lost pet

Make a PHOTO MONTAGE board that you can hang in your bedroom or somewhere at home. Ask mum or dad to help print your favourite photographs of you and your pet. Then attach them to a corkboard, which can be purchased at most stationery or department stores.

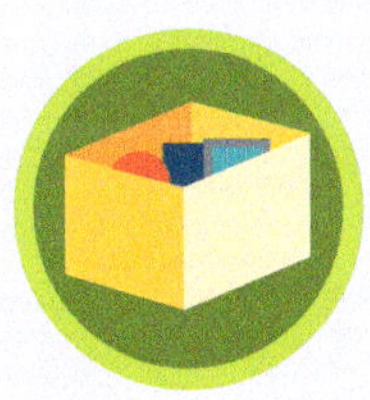

Make a KEEPSAKE BOX: Find a special box in a discount store that you can fill with precious memories of your pet. Then, when you have a particularly sad day, you could spend time quietly going through your memory box.

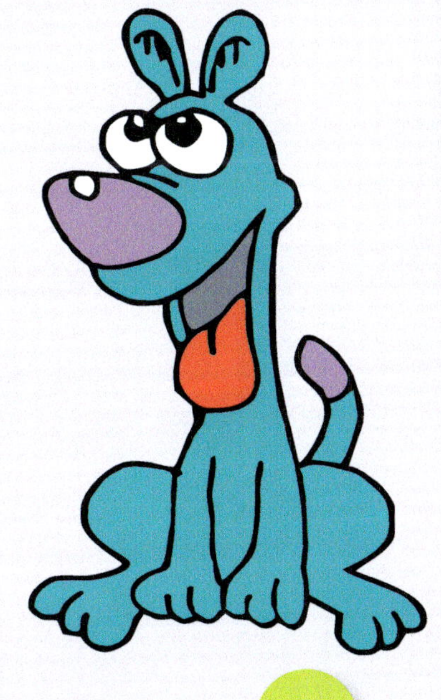

>>>

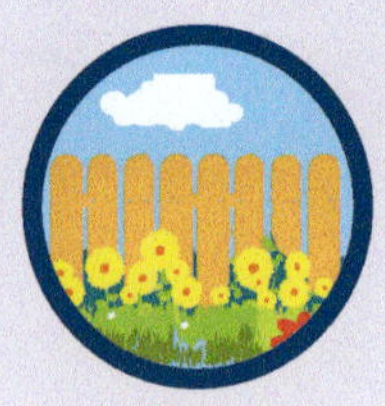

If you are able to bury your precious pet at home, you may like to set up a special MEMORIAL GARDEN to remember your pet. You may like to place the pet's special toys on that place and plant some beautiful flowers or a rose. Each spring, you can pick those flowers or roses to bring inside and remember your pet.

TALK with others about your beloved pet. Share funny stories and happy memories that you shared with your pet to keep the memories alive.

Get a FRAME and put a PHOTO of your pet in it. You might even have a photo of you and your pet to use. Then paint or decorate the frame.

Make up a SCRAPBOOK/ ALBUM of the happiest memories that you shared with your pet.

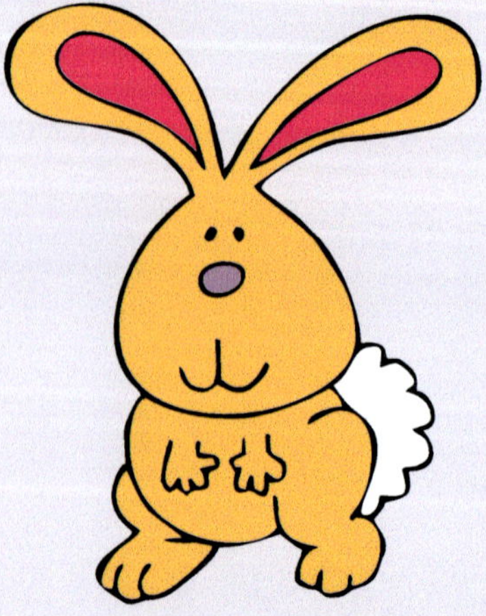

Parents

RELATING to your parents can be one of the most difficult parts of growing up. Trust me when I say that I can speak from experience on this one.

When you are getting older, especially as you are becoming a young man, your HORMONES can feel like they are out of control as your body changes. You have a strong desire to gain new independence. And on top of all this, your parents are trying to cope with your changes.

I have to say that parents are not perfect, but they are not meant to be. They do not have superhuman strength and knowledge. They are just adults who have teenagers for whom they are responsible. And they are often doing their best. Now, maybe they are doing a lousy job – in your opinion – but just remember that your parents are human.

It wasn't until I had my children that I realised what an amazing job parents do, and the incredible sacrifices they make just to keep us safe and happy.

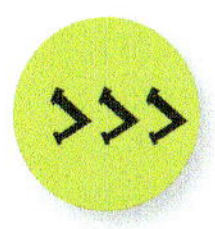

Your parents set up rules and boundaries for you – not to be meanspirited – but because they have more LIFE EXPERIENCE than you. They know what dangers and temptations are 'out there' in the wider world.

As you get older, your parents will gradually start to loosen those boundaries and you can begin to show them that you are growing up and taking more responsibility. But remember, your parents are basically acting out of CAUTION for much of the time, not wanting you to be hurt by others or by your actions. Whatever you believe to be true, your parents truly want the best for you.

'Children, obey your parents in the Lord, for this is right. "Honour your father and mother" which is the first commandment with a promise "so that it may go well with you and that you may enjoy long life on the earth."'

Ephesians 6: 1-3 (NIV)

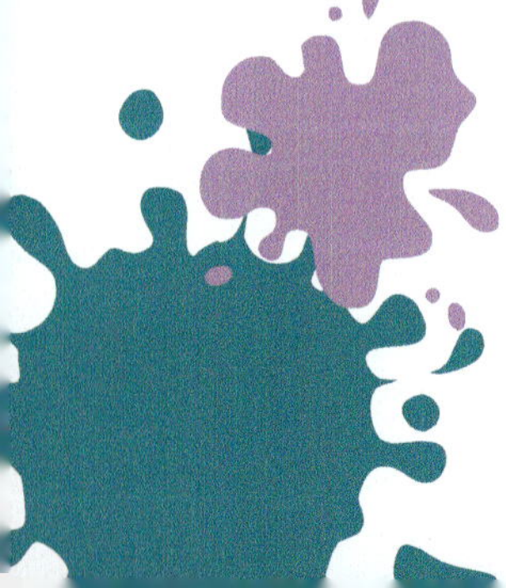

Sibling rivalry

Families can have their downsides. You may think that the real downers are the BROTHERS and SISTERS that your parents put under the same roof with you.

We can feel like our siblings were created with a prime directive to destroy our day and make life a constant misery. We can also often feel that WE are blamed for any misunderstandings and fights rather than our siblings, particularly if you are the older child.

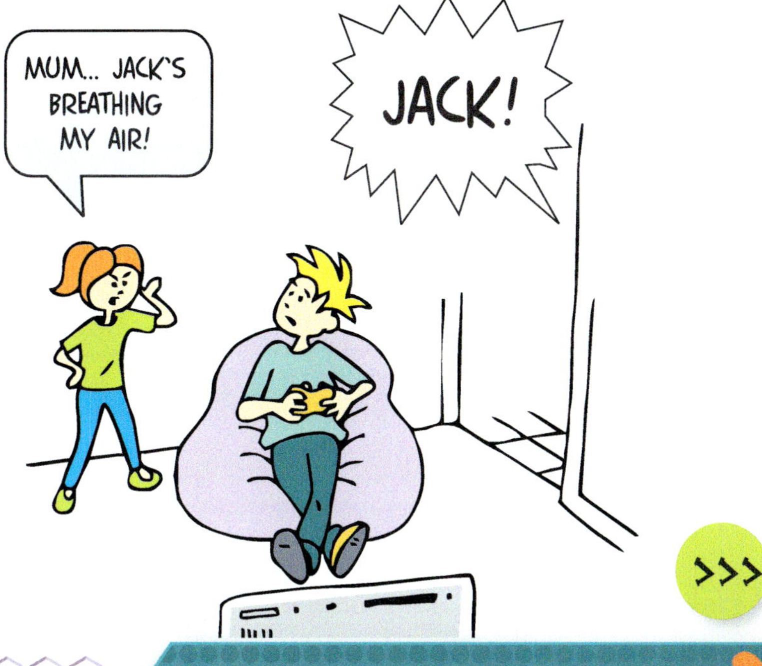

>>>

When I was young, there were many times when I was BLAMED for arguments with my younger brother. It seemed to be especially so because I was the older one and 'ought to have known better'!

If you feel constantly taunted or upset by family dynamics, chat with your parents about how you are feeling. (It is best to choose a time when everyone is calm; not in the middle of a screaming match!) Living within a family – particularly with siblings – is just a part of learning to RELATE TO OTHERS. In fact, those skills that you learn will help you to develop and maintain relationships.

Just think that when you are in the workforce in a few years time, you will not get to choose the people you will work alongside. Some colleagues will, most likely, be very different from you and may handle conflict in different ways to you. Learning to live in a family environment will PREPARE YOU, therefore, to deal with many other challenges in life.

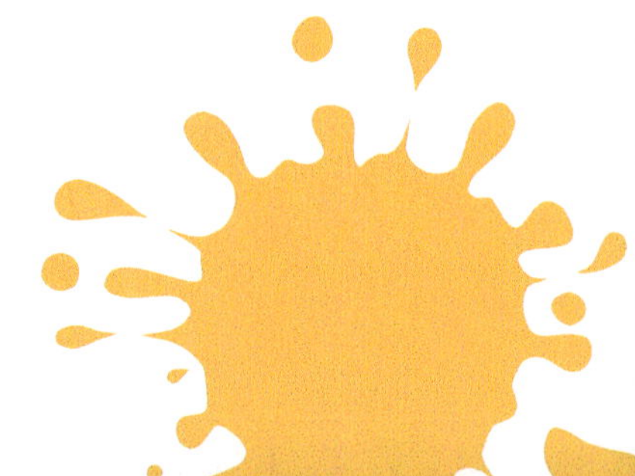

Eldest child syndrome

It's hard being the eldest

There is no doubt that being the eldest child can seem unfair.

I learnt – being the eldest of two children – that the oldest ones in the family PAVE THE WAY for younger siblings. That means that it is YOU who will probably experience the strictest rulings from parents. I know that it seems unfair to be the subject of parents' experiments with setting boundaries.

Curfews, bed times, movie choices, sleepovers: by the time your younger brothers or sisters get to your age, all the hard work and dramas with parents should be over.

I remember being 14 years-old. Being the eldest, I wasn't permitted to do a great deal of 'independent teenager' activities. Everyone in my class was invited to a birthday party in a town about half-an-hour's train ride away. Everyone in my class was allowed to travel by train on the Friday after school; that is, everyone EXCEPT ME!

I just could not understand why mum said 'no.' Everyone else was allowed to travel on the train together to attend

>>>

the party. We discussed it, but mum wouldn't budge. Either she was going to drive me to the party or I would not go! I agreed. I went and had a great time.

Eventually, when I began university, aged 17, I was allowed to finally travel on the train ALL BY MYSELF!

Another thing that really annoyed me about being the eldest, was that I was always blamed for EVERYTHING (well at least it seemed like that at the time!) Whenever I had problems with my younger brother, I seemed to be at fault. 'You should know better,' I remember being told. Though unfair at times, I got over it and forgave them. That's your challenge too. Understand what your parents are trying to do, and how much they love you. If you can't think about that at the time, reflect on it later.

So try to enjoy being the eldest, if you can. Just remember that you will have your driver's licence FIRST and will be able to go out on weekends BEFORE your younger siblings. That will be hard for them to handle. You will be able to move out of home first and come home to visit your family.

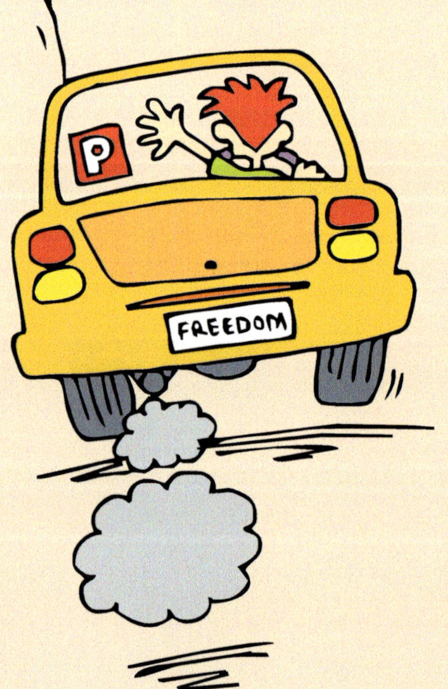

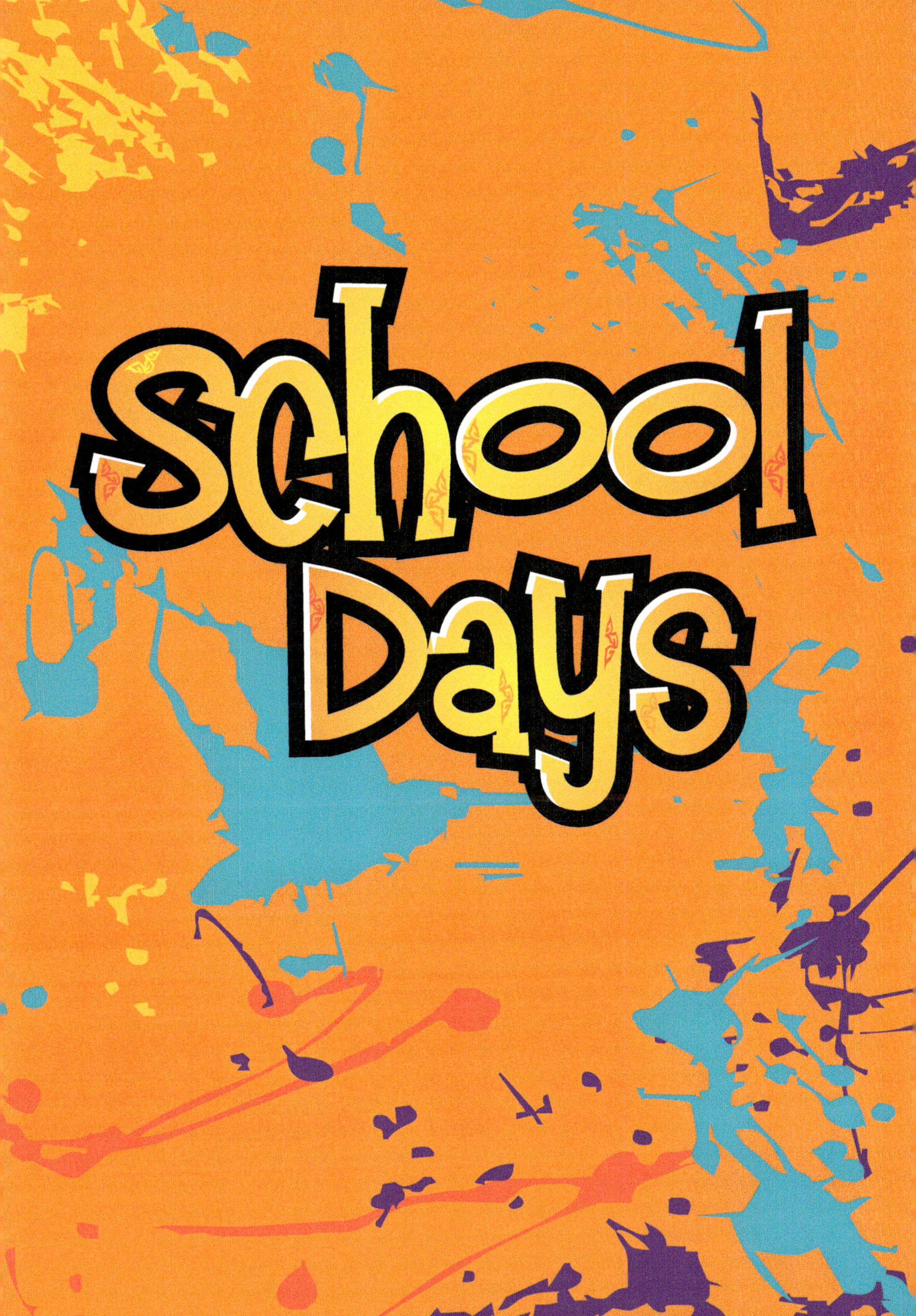
School Days

School life

Let's face it: going to school each day is a BIG part of life, and it goes over a number of years rather than one season or period of time. Right now, you are most probably in primary school, or perhaps you have just begun secondary school.

For some guys, school seems to come EASY. They love the social side of being at school for five days a week alongside mates, the chance to get outside at recess breaks and play basketball or kick a footy, while learning new ideas and concepts. You also get to complete interesting projects and work with a variety of people.

For some boys, however, school can have its CHALLENGES!

Maybe you have a learning problem that makes some subjects a little more difficult to learn. Or perhaps you find it a challenge to make new friends and find yourself spending a lot of time by yourself.

Hopefully, if that has been a problem for you, some of the following TIPS and STRATEGIES will help you feel more settled.

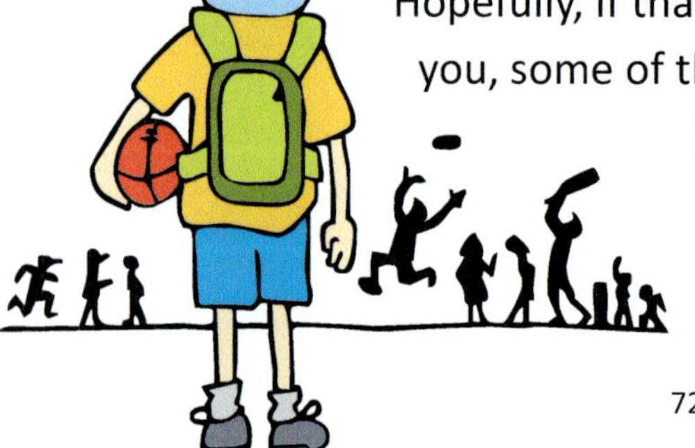

Settling into a new school

If you have moved house recently or have had to move schools for any other reason, it can be SCARY to start again at a new school. We can feel NERVOUS or WORRIED – even EXCITED – because we are UNSURE about what to expect.

'Will I make new friends easily?'
'Will I like my teachers, and will they like me?'
'Will I be able to find my way around the new school?'
'What if the work is much harder than I'm used to?'

These are all NORMAL questions to ponder when experiencing such a change.

Perhaps you know someone who already attends that school. Ask your mum or dad to help organise a time to catch up with them. You might be able to ask your friend some questions about your new school.

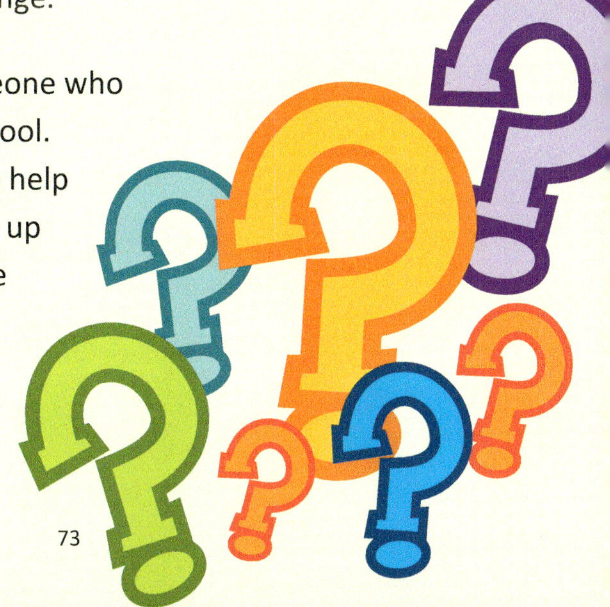

Tips for starting at your new school

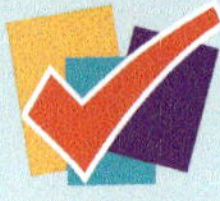

Make sure you have all the correct BOOKS and STATIONERY that you will need for your first day.

Ensure that all your books and stationery are LABELLED clearly.

Have a clean LUNCH BOX and plan some healthy snacks for during the day.

Pack a WATER BOTTLE.

Ask if you can have a MAP of the school, and highlight where your classroom is.

Find out the name of the person you need to MEET when you first arrive at school, and where to find that person.

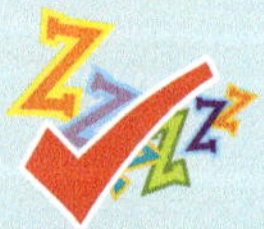

Make sure that you get to BED early the night before you start and have a good night's sleep.

Getting organised

Being organised is not a skill that comes easily to many boys. There's nothing wrong with that. In fact, for many children, being organised is not a natural concept. You may have a bedroom that is completely disorganised to a casual observer. Your clothes might be lying all over your 'FLOORDROBE' and the contents of your school bag all over your bed. But to YOU, it may be absolutely FINE! That's because YOU know where everything is *(well, mostly).*

But here's the deal: you actually need to keep your things in some sort of order, otherwise you are likely to misplace items that are REALLY important to you, or throw things out by mistake.

Imagine walking into a doctor's surgery, then having to step over a pile of papers, books, rubbish and clothes, just to reach the examination chair. I guess you would get the impression the doctor was not too serious about being a medical PROFESSIONAL. You would probably wonder what kind of doctor that person was!

In life, we need to have some sort of system to get ORGANISED, otherwise we tend to feel out of control and not sure what to do next. You can tell a lot about a person by the state of his/her bedroom at home. If there is chaos everywhere, the chances are that that person also feels life is pretty hectic and confusing. And organisation is generally NOT something that comes terribly easy for boys. For some, it does. But for many... well, let's just say that they are happy to live with the mess!

You can begin to organise your life better TODAY. You can start by organising your bedroom at home. Set aside an afternoon *(or a whole week if it's that bad)* to find homes for all your possessions. You can ask mum or dad to buy inexpensive BOXES or plastic containers from a local discount shop, or even some old shoeboxes. Then start labelling.

Make sure you label your boxes clearly so you will know where to find things when you need them.

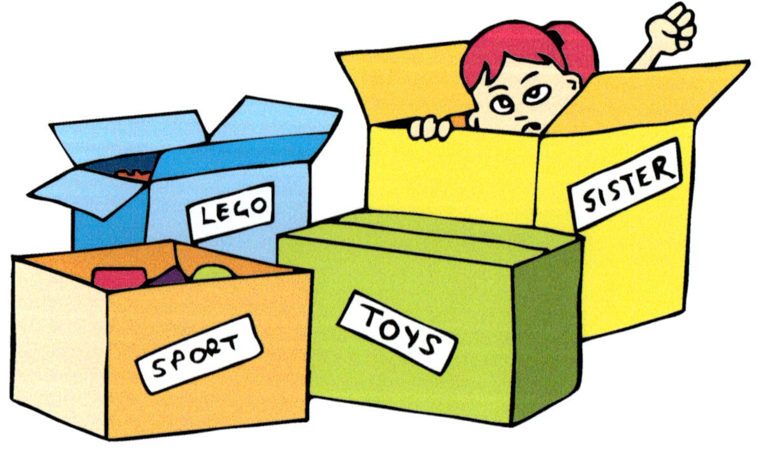

Things that you can organise into boxes

Photographs
School projects
CDs and discs
Letters
Action Figures
Keepsakes
Sports Cards
Badges

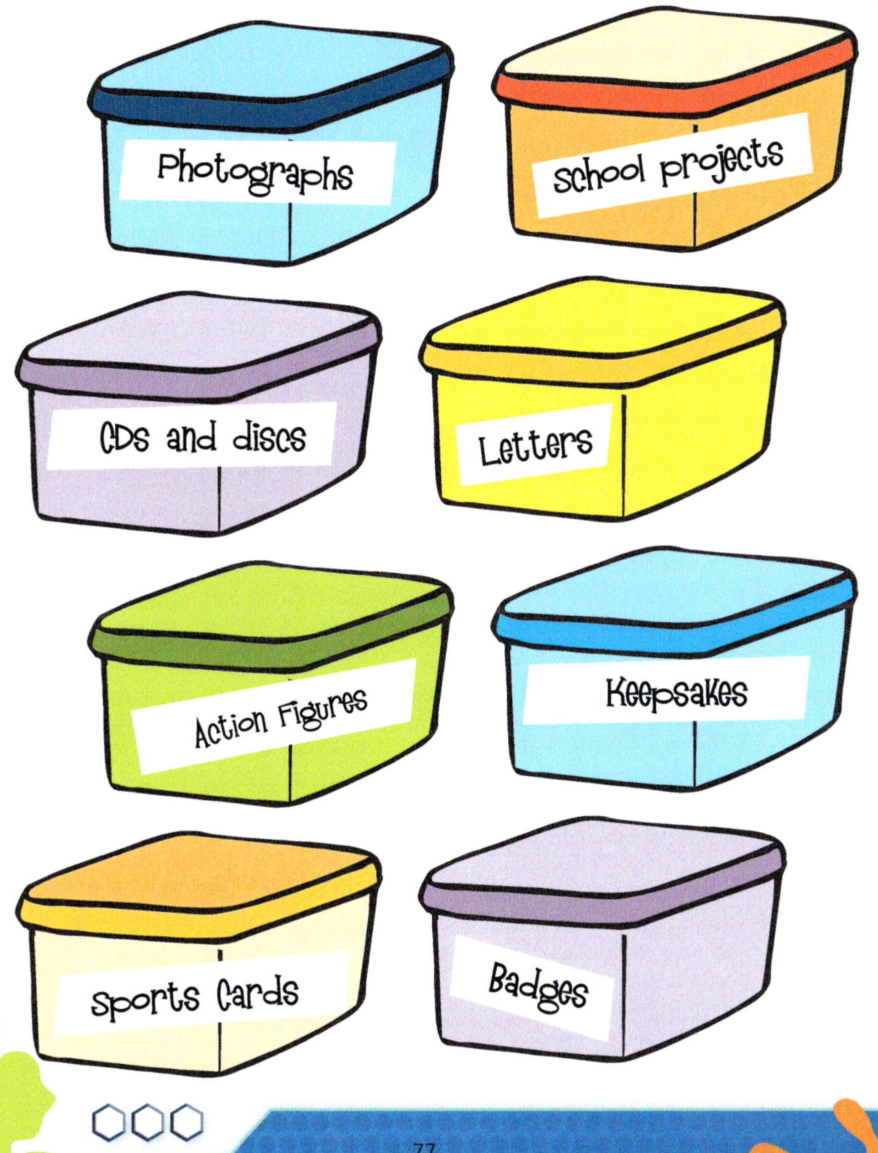

Getting started on the 'organised' you

You will feel so much BETTER once you begin to organise YOURSELF.

Some people do not have this as a natural gift in their lives, finding it difficult to organise things. It can seem like such a huge job that's scary to start.

Why not ask your family or a couple of close friends to HELP you out for a day?

Get yourself a cool diary. Diaries are NOT just for girls! If you don't have one already, get yourself a useful, simple diary. This is one of the best tools to help you get organised, especially for school. You can use different coloured markers to label homework subjects and set assignments. As you complete tasks, tick off what you complete.

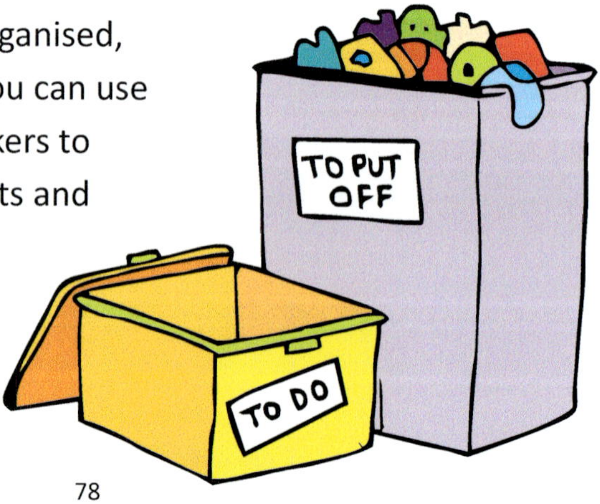

Friends & Mates

Friendships

Friendships are a BIG part of our lives and a God-given gift. Without our buddies, we could be left feeling very lonely and miserable. Friends help us feel like a part of a community: connected, loved and cared for.

You will form some friendships during primary school, and others well before. You may have some friends that you are related to – such as your cousins – or you may have met them at your sporting club or music class.

Perhaps you find making new friends easy, perhaps you find it difficult. If you don't seem to make friends easily, don't worry.

The following are some helpful tips and strategies that might help you build new friendships.

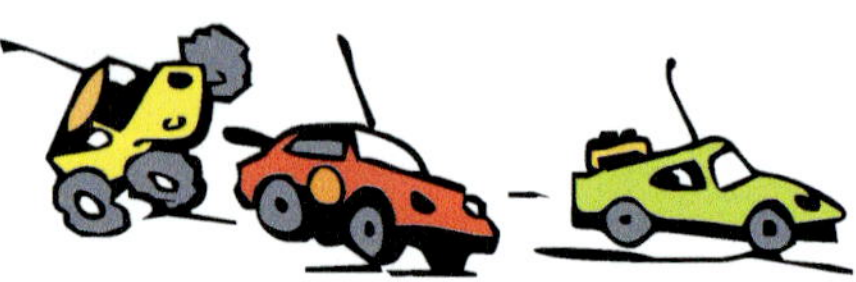

Friendships don't just happen, or do they?

'In order to make a friend, you have to be one first.'

Elbert Hubbard[9]

Think of your three closest mates for a minute.

Do you remember where you first met them and how you became friends?

My son's best mate is someone he met as a baby at a mother's group that I took him to. Those boys have now been buddies since they were 6 weeks-old. Okay, so they don't remember lying on a rug together on the floor drinking from baby bottles, but that's how long they've been hanging out together. They are still the BEST of mates 18 years later!

My son's other close friends have come from preschool days. Some met during school years, and others in sport.

>>>

One of my closest friendships came from someone I met at my work place. Right from the beginning, we just made each other laugh, and laugh! It has always felt like the chats and laughs have come so easy. Above all, we totally RESPECT each other. That means, even if we DISAGREE about something the other says, we remain friends.

Other friends I have formed over the years have come from living in the same street. We are all very close to our neighbours in a quiet court. Almost every day, I'll see a neighbour and say 'Hi.' Many times, we've gone beyond the odd 'Hello' to find out what's happening in people's lives. The more we talk, we more we form friendships.

I've made many other friends along the way just by being INTERESTED in others, SMILING when I meet someone new and ASKING QUESTIONS to get to know them better.

It doesn't take much to SAY HELLO to someone you haven't met before, but I am so glad I have done this on many occasions. If I hadn't tried talking with people, I would have missed out on some pretty awesome friendships!

Think about your five closest buddies... describe their personalities

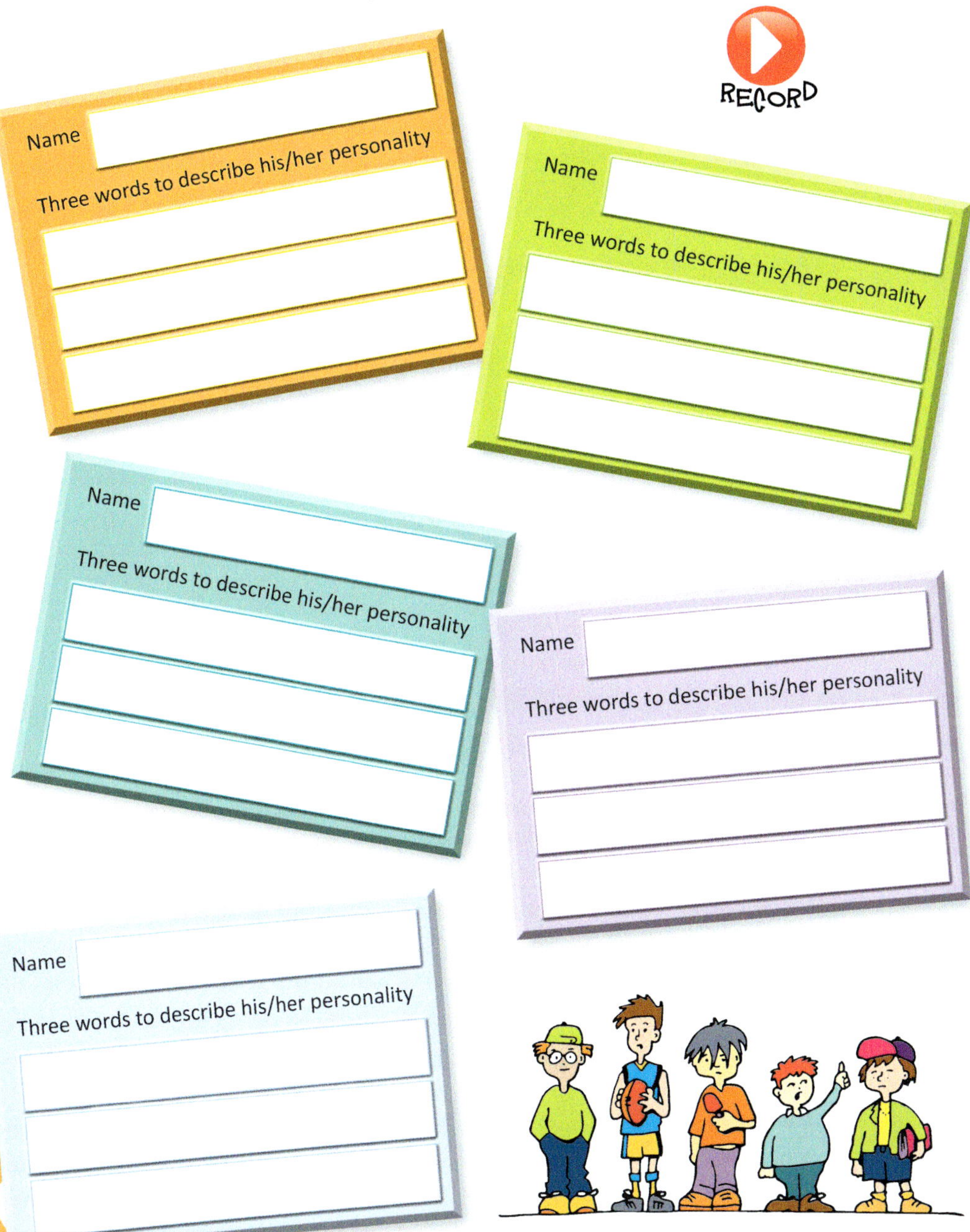

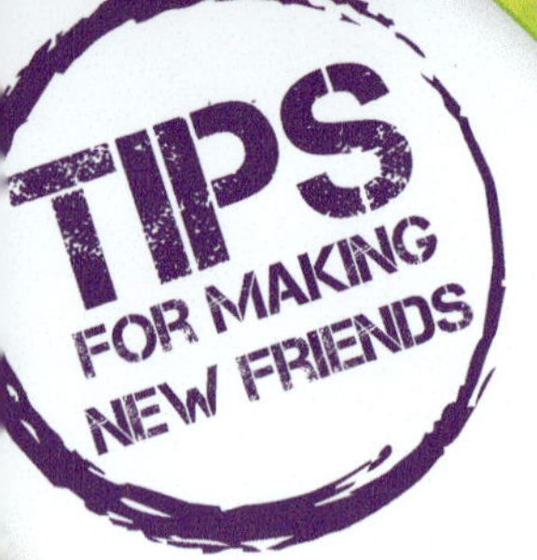

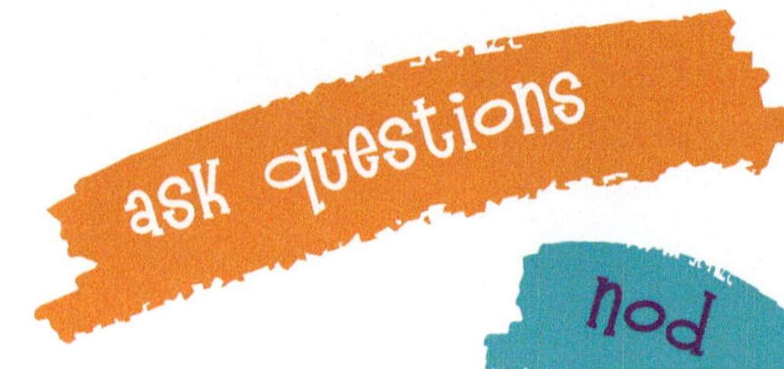

Be interested

Try to begin a conversation with someone new by showing that you are interested in THEM. If they are new to your school, you might begin by asking what school they came from, what they like to do for fun or how many family members they have. Once you begin asking questions, you're sure to find something in common to talk about.

Use eye contact

This probably seems like something SO SIMPLE but it's something that many people forget. Even before you first go up to a person and begin a conversation, use eye contact. Also make sure you nod, smile and look at them when you speak. There is nothing more off-putting than having a conversation with someone who spends half the time looking somewhere else, as if looking for someone or something far more interesting.

It's important to note, though, that there may be some cultures where this is not quite the same. But as a general rule, show interest in the person you're talking with, however that is best expressed.

Smile

Smile

A simple smile says SO MUCH. It says that you are willing to make a new friend. It says that you are happy to talk with the other person. It says that you are interested in getting to know them and that they are IMPORTANT! Most importantly, a smile costs you ABSOLUTELY NOTHING! Come to think of it, you have a never-ending supply of smiles available, so make sure you use them HEAPS!

be yourself

Be yourself

The best advice you can ever follow is to BE YOURSELF. No one else can be YOU, and YOU bring something to your friendship groups that no one else does.

Sometimes, there are very real pressures to try and act like others. It is easy to think your personality is boring and uninteresting. But that's not being real. The problem with not being yourself when you first make a new friend is that you have to keep up appearances. That means, if you PRETEND that you REALLY LIKE riding motorbikes, pretty soon your mates will want to go riding with you because it's something that you said YOU enjoy. Or maybe you SAY that you love skateboarding.

>>>

TIPS
FOR MAKING
NEW FRIENDS

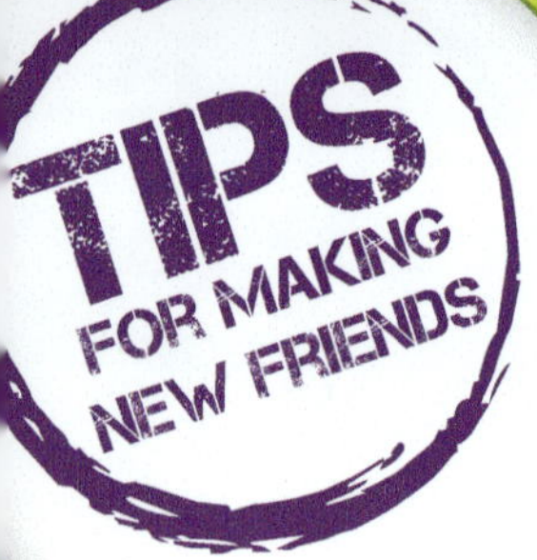

Before you know it, your new mates will be asking you to dig out that skateboard of yours (even if it doesn't exist) and hit the ramps.

Just stop! The real you is fine, and worth getting to know, even if your real hobby is collecting volcanic rocks. ☺

real you

Ask questions

When you first meet and get to know a new friend – or haven't seen them in a while – make sure you ask lots of QUESTIONS. Sure, it's great to share YOUR stories and interests, but make sure you also ask questions to get to know the other person.

MATE, WE HAVEN'T CAUGHT UP FOR AGES...
BE FRIENDS WITH ME ON FACEBOOK.

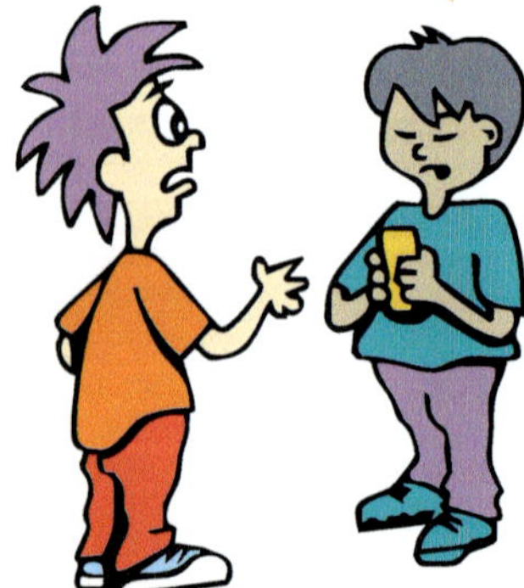

Have a look at the next page for some ideas.

conversation

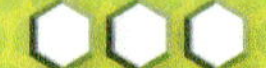

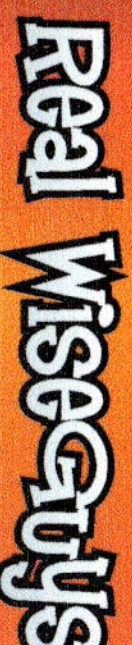

Home Connect

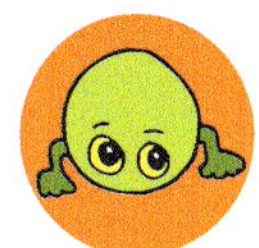

Seth, age 9

'If someone is feeling sad because he is new to the school, try inviting him to join in your game. He might just be feeling shy.'

Home Connect

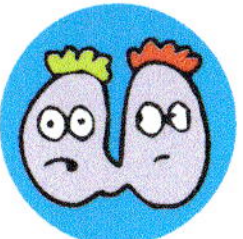

Jay, aged 11

'Be yourself. Always be nice and play games others like, not just the games you like.'

Home Connect

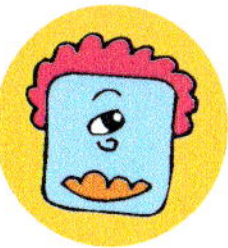

Zavier, age 10

'Be nice to others and they'll usually be nice back. Show respect and kindness.'

Home Connect

Will, age 6

'If you want to make a new friend, sometimes you have to play his game, not just your game. And you have to be nice!'

Home Connect

Search

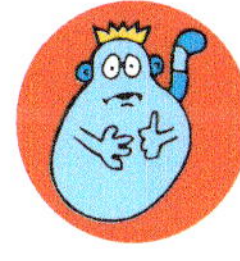

Jackson, age 8

'To make a friend, you need to be nice. Let others play your games (like join in your handball game), give them some of your spare collectors cards (like animal or sports ones). Once you are friends, invite them over for a play.'

Home Connect

Jesse, age 8

'Be nice to others and ask them questions. Ask them if they want to join in your game or sit at your table in class.'

Home Connect

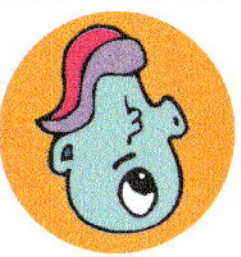

Jake, age 9

'If someone looks lonely or he doesn't seem to be playing with someone else, ask him to join in your game. He might just be shy.'

Friendship icebreakers

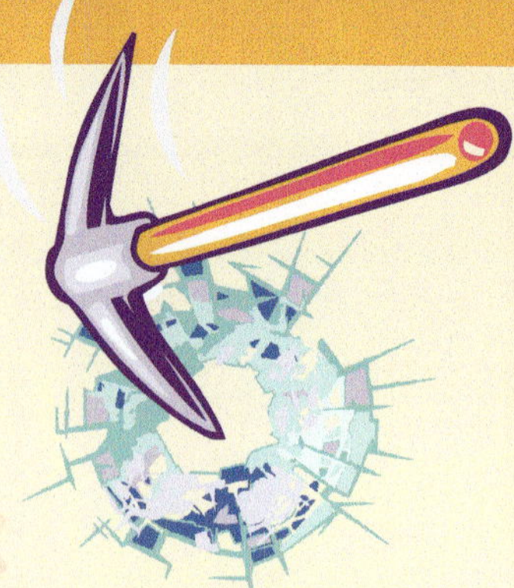

Questions you can ask a new friend...

How many people are in your family?

What is the strangest/funniest pet you've owned?

How many schools have you attended?

If you could have an entire day to do anything you wanted, what would you do?

Is there a sports team, or athlete, you support?

Do you play a musical instrument?

Have you ever travelled overseas?

What is your favourite colour?

What is the weirdest gift you have ever received?

Are you scared of any animals or insects?

What is your favourite television show?

If you had a super power, what would you want and why?

Who do you admire most and why?

What was your favourite birthday you have had and what made it so special?

Is there a pet you wish you could own but your parents won't let you?

What would you change about yourself and why?

Do you have any strange habits?

What special talents do you have?

Do you go to church?

What do you want to do when you grow up?

What is your favourite thing to do on a rainy day?

Who is your favourite band/music artist?

What is your all-time favourite movie?

Rights of a friend

Having friends is a great RESPONSIBILITY. As we've already discussed, being a friend to someone means that you have to put in some work. It shouldn't always be hard work, which we'll talk about later. But all friends should get some basic things right. What I've written below are qualities and actions that you should expect and deserve from a friend.

'Many people will walk in and out of your life, But only true friends will leave footprints in your heart.'

Eleanor Roosevelt

Trust

You should be able to trust a real friend. You should expect that they will keep things you tell them PRIVATE, especially if it is something very personal that you don't want the whole world knowing about. If they do share your secrets with others, you need to let your friend know that it is not okay. ***(By the way, there may be times when you need to tell a friend's secret to an adult if you***

are worried about his health or if someone is hurting him. Talk to your parent or guardian about times like these so you know what to do if it ever happens.)

Care

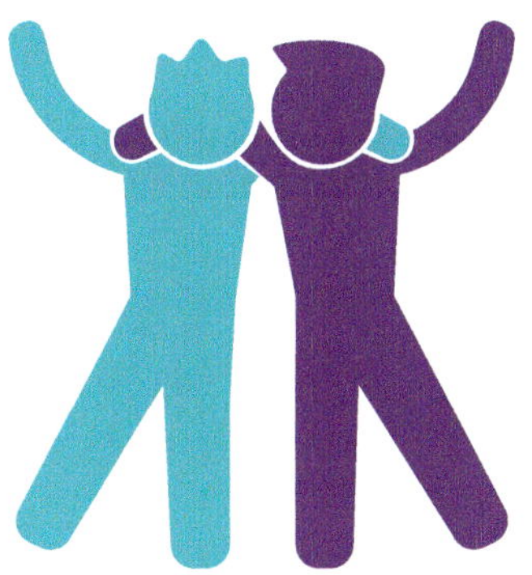

Your friend should always show that they care about your WELFARE – how you are going right now – and your feelings. If a friend is nasty to your face or behind your back, you have a right to let them know that you feel hurt.

Respect

A true friend should always show respect to you and your belongings. For example, a friend should not simply go through your pencil case at school just because you are his friend and probably wouldn't mind. A friend still respects you enough to ask first. A friend also respects you in the way he TALKS TO you and ABOUT YOU to others.

And YOUR friends should be able to expect the SAME from you in return.

Dealing with shyness

Many boys are shy. It will feel like your heart is nearly leaping out of your chest at the very thought of being put in a new situation or being confronted with having to make new friends. Being shy is nothing to be embarrassed or worried about. MANY kids, and adults, feel this way and get through life just fine.

But if you struggle with feeling shy, here are a few tips to help you make some friends.

Expect others to like you

When you feel shy, you can also feel like people might not want to talk with you or may not like you. Forget about feeling like that. When you are meeting new people, go into it with an attitude that they WILL like you.

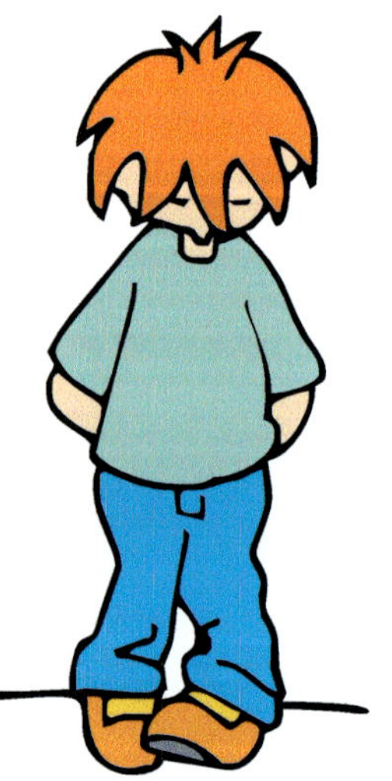

Think of five questions that you could ask a new person you meet

The list we looked at before gives you some ideas for 'breaking the ice' when it comes to conversations. Questions like those, or the simple first-up ones below, give you some ideas before you are actually faced with a situation in which you may have to talk. So think up some prepared questions first.

Here are a few ideas to help you:

Where do you live?

How many people make up your family?

Who is your favourite singer or band?

What school do you go to, or have been to in the past?

What are your favourite hobbies / sports?

Practise in front of a mirror

If you are REALLY shy, you might want to practise asking these questions in front of a mirror and watch what your face is doing when you talk. For example, make sure you are SMILING when you ask these questions. Your smiling face will actually help you to relax and will also be a welcoming gesture to the person you are talking to.

Remember, a smile instantly puts two people at ease.

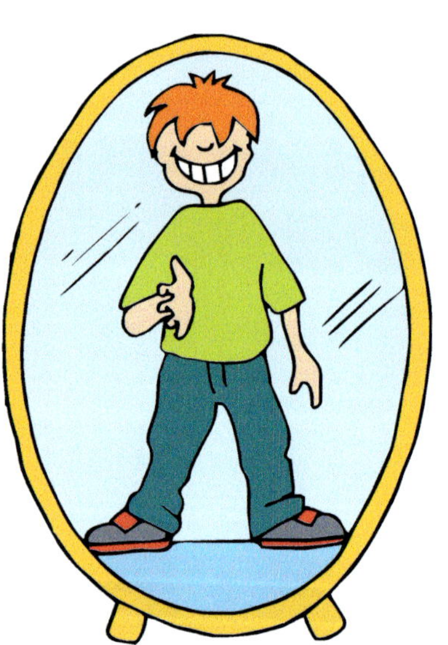

You could also practise talking with a family member at home. Ask them for feedback.

Relax

Take the time to relax before you go into a new situation. Take 5-10 very deep breaths; put yourself in a positive frame of mind and SMILE. A smile is a way to relax instantly.

Pray

Ask God to bring a special friend into your life, perhaps one you haven't met yet.

When friendships are NO fun!

Friendships that are NOT too healthy for you!

Unhealthy friendships can feel a bit like a vacuum cleaner sucking all the energy out of you. These friendships can feel totally one-sided. That means that one person is always doing all the work and having to work at the friendship.

'There are "friends" who destroy each other, but a real friend sticks closer than a brother.'

Proverbs 18:24 (NLT)

Sure, it's true that all great friendships will be tested at times, but it's important to remember that it should work like a true partnership. In simple words, it needs to work for BOTH of you.

Needy friends can be quite difficult – the friend who has a low self-image may often complain that they are 'stupid' or 'too ugly' or 'nobody likes me'.

>>>

My advice for supporting a friend like this is to tell your friend they are important and VALUED. Try not to comment on phrases like... 'I'm stupid', or 'I'm ugly'.

If you begin to get worried about a friend's health, of course, MAKE SURE YOU TELL AN ADULT. But otherwise, try to ignore negative behaviour, as it will only bring you down too, and you don't need that.

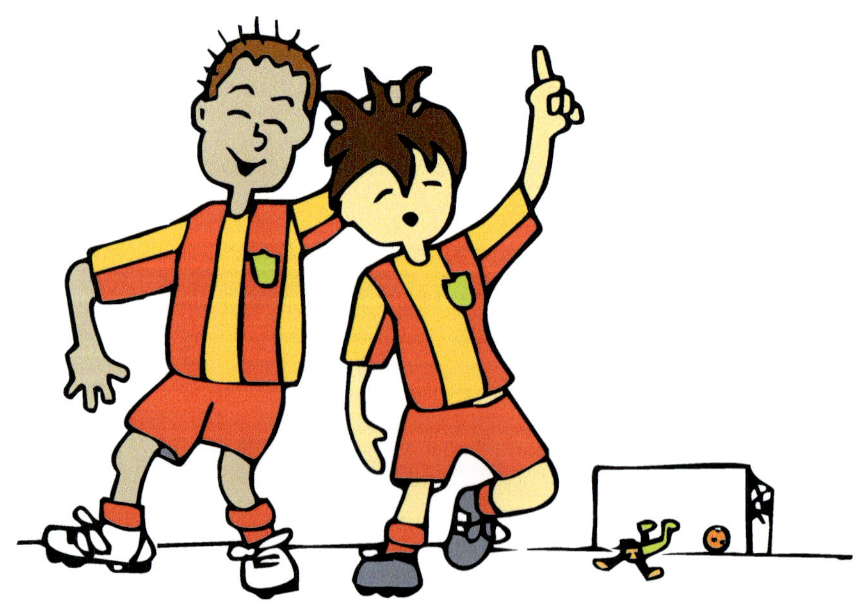

Peer pressure

Peer pressure is basically feeling pushed to do something that you don't feel comfortable about.

'Escape quickly from the company of fools; they're a waste of your time, a waste of your words.'
Proverbs 14:7 (The Message)

Imagine this scene from a playground: two kids tell you to throw a stone at another boy. This is one example of peer pressure and you have a choice to make: to throw, or not throw?

As you go through primary school, the choices that you face might become a little more advanced, like whether to follow your friends and go out of bounds during recess.

Decide now, that you'll always choose the best decision for YOU no matter what. That way, it won't be so difficult when you face the pressure to do something that you're not comfortable with.

How do I know what the right decision is?

We all have an inbuilt system that helps us when we are faced with a difficult decision to make. It is called your INTUITION.

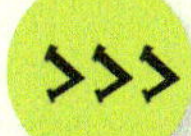

Your intuition is that feeling in your stomach that helps you know whether a situation is right or not. It also helps you to make the correct decision. For example, a mate might ask you to go to the teacher's desk drawer and grab a pen. You know, deep down inside, that you aren't supposed to open the teacher's drawer without asking.

When you THINK about going up to the teacher's desk, opening the drawer and taking a pen, you actually feel uneasy and a bit sick in your stomach. You might even have a picture in your mind of your teacher's disappointed face. THAT is your intuition, your inner voice telling you that it isn't the right decision.

If you are not sure whether you are about to make the right decision or not, try this: imagine that you have just made the decision to go up and take the pen without asking. *Really feel* what that would be like. Do you feel HAPPY and RELAXED? Are you NERVOUS and feeling GUILTY that you helped yourself without permission? Do you FEEL that you have done the wrong thing?

Once you have thought about what this feels like, you should have a fairly good idea of what decision you should make.

'Become wise by walking with the wise; hang out with fools and watch your life fall to pieces.'
Proverbs 13:20 The Message

Talking Friends

Home Connect 

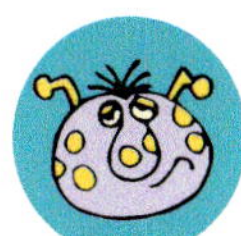

Aiden, age 8

I enjoy hanging out with my mates. We usually ride our bikes together after school or build cubbies. We enjoy doing fun stuff together.

Home Connect 

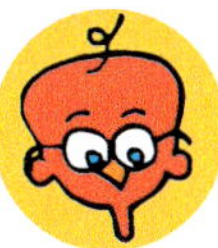

Ben, age 10

I haven't always made friends easily. It can be really hard sometimes to go up to someone you don't know and ask if you can play with them. But usually, they say 'yes' and you've made another friend just by asking. So sometimes, you just have to get out there and ask!

Home Connect 

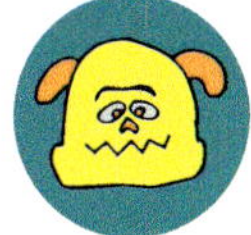

Jacob, age 9

I have been mates with my best friend Jake, since we were in Kindergarten together. Our Mums are good friends and I like that we get to celebrate our birthdays together. We like playing games together on the computer.

Home Connect

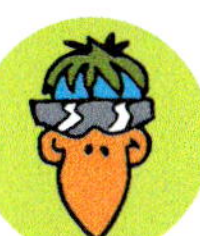

Jamie, age 7

When I first started at my new school I was fairly shy and didn't know who I should play with. But after a few weeks, I got to know a few of the boys in my class and we started playing at recess.

Home Connect 

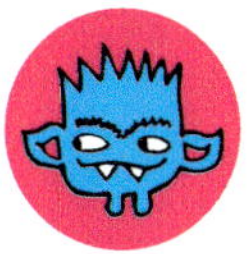

Cameron, age 10

I am really thankful for my friends. I enjoy hanging out with them at school and on the weekend. One time, our Dads even took us camping for the whole weekend. We had so much fun and got really muddy!

Home Connect 

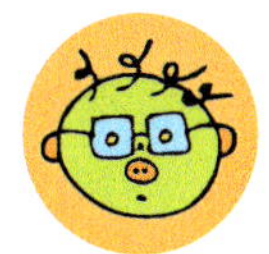

Billie, age 11

You need to remember to be friendly towards others because sometimes people can be really shy. Go up to someone who seems lonely and ask them to hang out with you at recess. You never know – you might make a new friend.

What does a great friend look like?

Write all of the qualities that you appreciate in your friends.

RECORD ....

....

....

....

....

....

'True friends will be there with you to share the giggles in the good times and cry with you in the bad times.'

Anonymous

Bullying & Clashes

Bullying: it hurts in so many ways

For whatever reason, some kids treat others unkindly. When someone chooses to be unkind or bully another person, it will more likely reveal a lot more about THAT person than it does about the one targeted.

Someone who threatens, teases, behaves nastily or makes others feel small, is most often struggling with his or her own thoughts of being sad, alone, unloved or having a poor self image. If the bully makes others feel small and inadequate, perhaps he or she will feel bigger and even more important. Bullying others doesn't work that way. The bully ends up looking unkind, small and just plain nasty.

Bullying – physical and emotional

It may not be physical bullying that you experience, but EMOTIONAL bullying, such as being teased, talked about or deliberately left out of games or conversations. This can hurt just as much.

What is bullying?

Bullying can include the following:

- Hurting someone physically, such as hitting or pushing
- Name-calling
- Deliberately excluding someone, or leaving them out of activities
- Nasty talk, such as speaking behind someone's back or making up stories that are untrue

Usually, these behaviours become bullying when it happens CONSISTENTLY (occurring often or all of the time.)

It can feel like it is never going to stop and it can leave you feeling ANGRY, SAD, ALONE, CONFUSED, SCARED or DISTRESSED.

Tell someone who cares about you

Here are some things you can do if another child, or older person, is often causing you to feel small and sad.

Even if the person bullying you tells you NOT TO TELL ANYONE, you MUST tell a person you trust about what is happening to you. No one deserves to feel scared, intimidated or small because of how someone else is behaving.

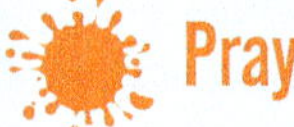

Pray

Pray for yourself. It can be as simple as saying secret words in your mind to God. Ask Him to help you be strong and brave, preventing a bully's actions from upsetting you further. Ask God to give you an extra measure of STRENGTH. Pray for the bully too. That person has a lot to learn about how to treat others with kindness and respect.

Ignore a bully

Bullies get their power only if YOU give it away. Reacting to bullies with anger actually gives them what they are after. Ignoring bullies takes away their bully powers and it all comes back to you.

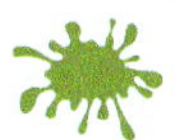

Say 'No!'

As soon as you say this single, powerful word – 'NO!' – you are letting bullies know, loud and clear, that what they are doing or saying is not okay. If you struggle a bit with this at first, start by saying it under your breath or in your mind until you soon have the courage to say it out loud, with authority. You are worth it! Saying 'No' also lets everyone else around you know that what is happening is not okay. They become witnesses to the bullying and your desire for it to stop.

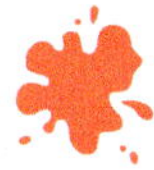

Stand tall and have confidence

Bullies are looking for people they can steal from. They want your confidence. And they only get it by taking yours. Try to remember that bullies are really just people who lack personal confidence. Bullies try to make others FEEL INFERIOR to hide their own insecurities. When you remember this fact, you realise bullies are just people who lack confidence.

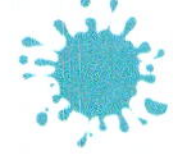

Don't look the other way if you see someone being bullied

If you see friends or others being bullied, you owe it to them to let someone know. Tell a teacher or your parents what is happening.

Need a bit more information or help?
Take a look at this website: **www.bullyingnoway.gov.au**

Dealing with bullies

Home Connect Search

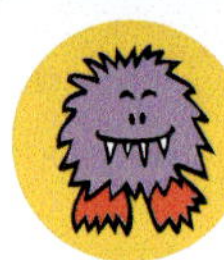

Name supplied, age 10

'I am in Year 5 at school and I have a problem with a couple of the boys in my year level. They aren't in the same grade as me but the problems really happen at recess and other break times. These couple of boys are a lot taller and bigger than me. They don't really ***ever talk*** to me, but every time they walk past me they give me a not-so-gentle nudge. It doesn't really hurt that much; it's more annoying. Every time I see them when I'm walking around the yard at school, I already know what they are going to do. Sometimes, they say sorry after they have nudged me, especially if they see others around, but I just know that it is deliberate because they do it every single time, and most days. I don't want to tell my mum or dad about it because I know my mum will go straight up to the school and I don't want it to get any worse when these boys find out I told on them. What do I do?'

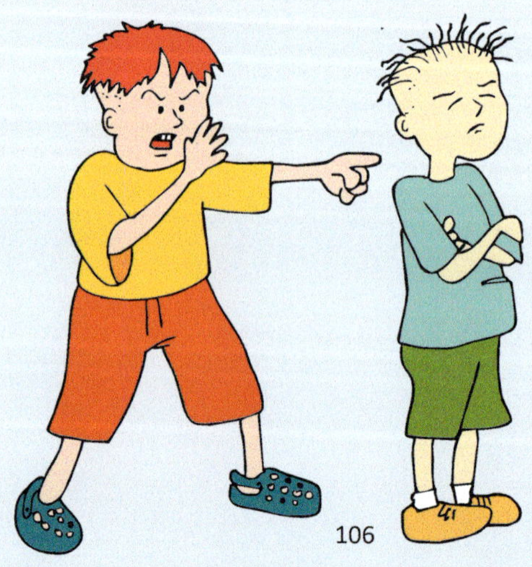

Hi there,

Firstly, this behaviour is totally NOT OKAY – not even close to okay! You have every right to feel safe and secure at school at all times. The behaviour of these two boys is ensuring that this is not the case. You should be able to go out at break times, or anytime for that matter, at school without having to worry about being deliberately bumped or picked on. Have you tried actually saying the words, 'STOP IT!' to these boys? It's worth a try in a loud but firm voice next time they bump into you.

If the behaviour continues after this, you absolutely **need to tell a trusted adult about this behaviour.** I know you may feel really uncomfortable about this, but here's the thing: *How would you feel knowing that another boy may be going through exactly the same experience as you, or could face it in the future? What if this was your younger brother or sister? Would you want them to let someone know it was happening?*

This is bullying because it is DELIBERATE and REPEATED behaviour. And if they continue to get away with this, they will eventually move onto another target and repeat the same behaviour. Why? Because this type of behaviour helps them to feel bigger and more significant by making others (such as yourself) feel small.

Talk to your class teacher, mum or dad or any other adult that you feel comfortable with. This is NOT your problem to fix and you are NOT to blame. Often, we are scared to tell someone about being bullied because we might feel EMBARRASSED or HUMILIATED that we are being targeted. But it honestly could be anyone. So tell an adult and let them deal with the situation and help guide you through it. Bullying is NEVER okay!

Sharon

Thoughts in a jar

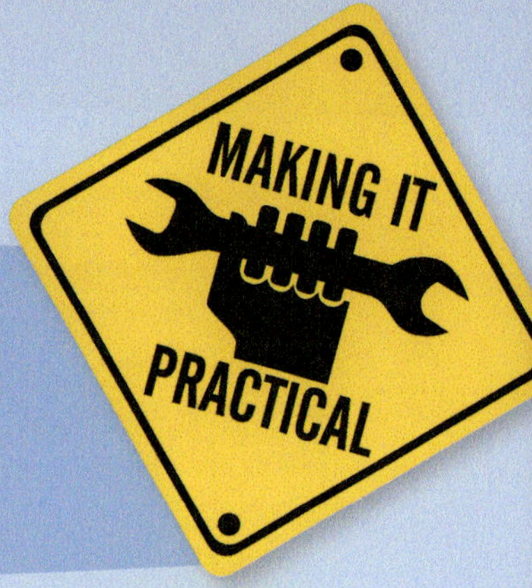

You will need:

- A glass or plastic jar or a small box, preferably with a lid
- A packet of coloured sticky notes
- Coloured pens or felt tip markers

Sometimes, we can have strong feelings, emotions and experiences. Often, they are still **BOTHERING US** at the end of a day. Someone may have said a rude or uncaring comment or you feel sad or bullied. Try this idea...

Write your thoughts and feelings down on a piece of paper.

Fold the piece of paper in half, and then halve again. Place into jar and place the lid back on.

Repeat this each day!

You may write positive things as well, or write a problem or situation that is troubling you.

Commit the jar thoughts to God. Ask God to deal with your problems for you.

Later on, go back and read through some of the notes. The anxious and sad feelings you wrote may become less intense. When reading those thoughts back later, you may feel more settled... or you can be happy to just keep the words sealed in that jar, safely hidden and without any power to harm you!

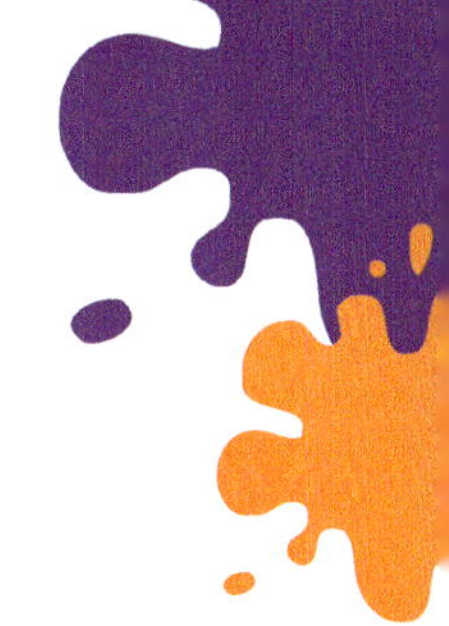

Sticks and stones

Name-calling is BULLYING. You may know the expression, *'Sticks and stones may break my bones but words will never harm me'.* This can be far from true!

I can recall vividly an example of verbal bullying, way back as a 12 year-old, while in Year 7. I have always been someone of small stature, and was easily the smallest in my class back then. One fellow student came up with the nickname 'weasel' for me.

I absolutely hated that. It made me feel like some awful little animal.

Why couldn't they think up a title like 'little cutie' or something like that?

Well, I coped pretty well despite the name-calling. Most times, I found a way of not letting it sit in my head.

Until, however, the last day of the school year when our class teacher was giving out Christmas cards. They were lovely hand-made cards with caricatures of each student on the front of every card. As mine came around, I couldn't believe my eyes – right there, above my very cute portrait, was the word **'Weasel'!** I couldn't believe that even my teacher had picked up on that name.

Well, I am still small in stature, but I don't let it bother me.

I tell this story to illustrate how names can stick with us if we don't do something about it. Some 25 years later, I can still recall that experience as though it happened yesterday. What I do today, though, is take away the power of those words by saying to myself, 'they are not true.'

You don't have to wait 25 years. You can do it today. Say it right now before reading on, and enjoy the power that YOU get back.

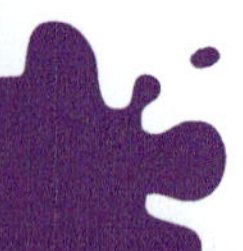

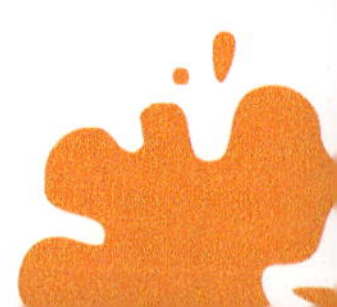

A clash of personalities

Sometimes, you will find that you are in a class at school or even within your sports team with someone who just annoys you. This can sometimes be a clash of personalities. For example, you may be a QUIET or SHY person and like to have peace and quiet around you. There might be a friend or family member around, however, who likes to be the centre of attention and is often LOUD and very VOCAL.

You might feel frustrated or even a little angry at how this person behaves. It might really, really annoy you.

But here's the thing: God has created EVERYONE as unique and different. Some are loud, energetic and always talk or give their opinions, while others are less talkative and like to listen to what others are saying – not voicing their opinions too often. That doesn't mean that they are terrible people. It just means that they are different to YOU.

Learning tolerance

As friends, we all need to learn TOLERANCE, because sometimes others may frustrate us by the way they behave. It can easily get us down. We all need to learn to tolerate others and their personalities. You can't always control who you will spend time with – whether that be team mates on your football or basketball team, or relatives at a big family barbecue. Sometimes, you need to smile and remember to be interested in what others have to say.

As a side note, being tolerant DOESN'T mean that you have to put up with behaviour that is UNACCEPTABLE, such as bullying, nasty remarks or physical threats. THIS IS NEVER OKAY. But just remember that one day you will be out in the big wide world working in a job, and you can't control the different personalities that you will work with. So learning to get along with others and accept that we are created different is a part of growing up.

***You cannot control others' behaviours, but you can always control* YOUR OWN.**

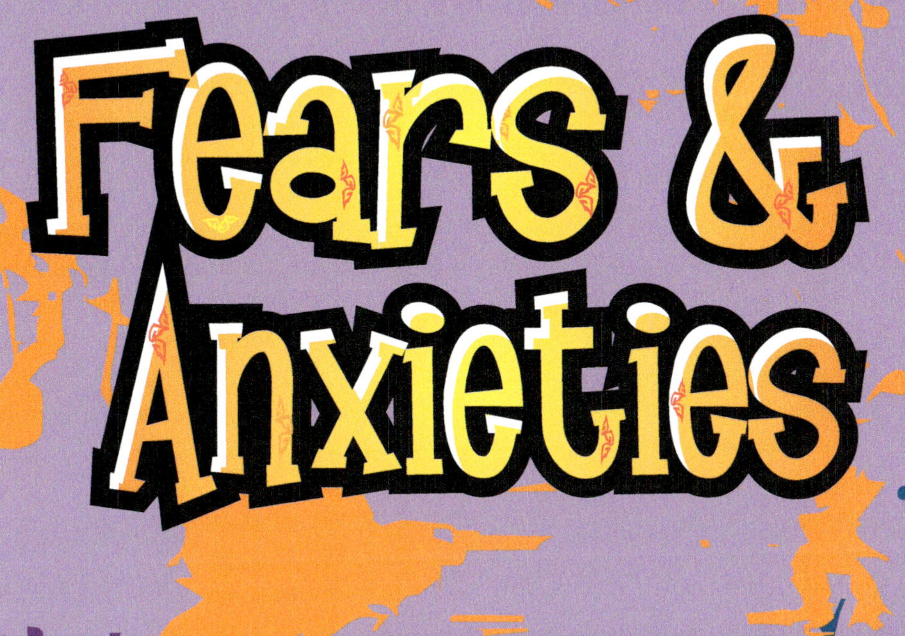
Fears &
Anxieties

Fears and anxieties

All of us experience fears and anxieties at different times. You might feel ANXIOUS when you face different and NEW situations that you haven't experienced before.

'Do not be anxious about anything, but in every situation, by prayer and petition, with thanksgiving, present your requests to God.'

Philippians 4:6 (NIV)

Situations that you might feel anxious about may include the following:

- **Starting a new school**
- **Visiting someone in hospital**
- **Going to the dentist**
- **Moving home**
- **Starting in a new sports team or music group**
- **Performing on stage**
- **Sitting a maths test**
- **Going to a party where you only know the host**
- **A sleepover at a friend's house**
- **Getting your tonsils taken out in hospital**
- **Performing in a school play**
- **Giving a speech in front of your class**
- **Having a new family member join you**
- **Playing in a basketball or football grand final**

Any of these situations might cause you to feel a little worried or anxious. These are perfectly NORMAL feelings. Everyone from famous celebrities about to step on stage, to doctors performing lifesaving surgery on a patient, all feel this way at times. When you face a new or different experience, you may feel any of the following:

- **Sensing fluttering sensations in your stomach**
- **Sickness, or an ache, in your stomach**
- **Sweating**
- **Dry mouth**
- **Headache**
- **Heart racing**
- **Shaking hands**

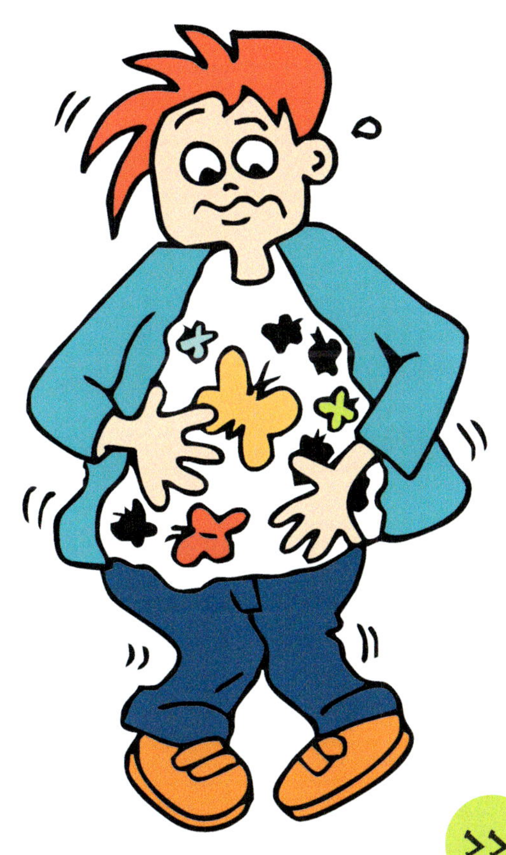

These are all symptoms that indicate that you are worried or NERVOUS. That is perfectly normal.

When we face new and different situations, we are often fearful of what will happen.

I remember a few years ago, when I was asked to first appear on a national television program. I felt very nervous and worried because I knew that there would be many thousands of people watching me live during the interview. My heart raced and it felt like there were thousands of little butterflies all having a party in my stomach.

I was very scared of things that MIGHT HAPPEN. I imagined all of the things that could possibly go WRONG on live television.

'What if I forget what I need to say?'

'I might freeze and not be able to speak!'

'What if I vomit live on air, all over the host sitting next to me?'

It's interesting how we think of all the horrible things that could happen, imagining our lives damaged by what may NEVER HAPPEN.

Your time is better spent focusing on all of the great things that might come out of our new experiences. For example, after I had been interviewed on live television, and realised that I was very comfortable being on camera, I was much better PREPARED and RELAXED the next time I had to do a TV interview.

Perhaps you have been asked to give a talk in front of your class. You may feel very WORRIED and NERVOUS about speaking in front of your peers. You may worry that you will forget all of the information you want to share. You may also be concerned that students won't be interested in what you have to say, or that you will stutter or freeze in front of the group. All of these things that you imagine might happen are just that – a part of your IMAGINATION. They haven't happened yet and are not likely to happen. But we can feed our nervousness by imagining that the worst events WILL happen.

You can change how your body reacts to a new situation by REPLACING your thoughts and attitudes about it.

Instead of thinking or saying, **'I CAN'T speak in front of my class. I cannot do it'**, try REPHRASING your thoughts to something positive: **'I have a great opportunity to share this (story or information) with my classmates. I will be confident and smile a lot.'**

"'For I know the plans I have for you,' declares the Lord, 'plans to prosper you and not to harm you, plans to give you hope and a future.'"

Jeremiah 29:11 (NIV)

Things you can do if you are feeling UNEASY or NERVOUS about a new situation

- Take long, deep breaths in and out.
- Have a good night's sleep the day before a new event, so that you are well rested.
- Go for a run or play a game of basketball; do anything physical to get your blood pumping through your body.
- Talk positively to yourself about the new experience. Don't think about the things that could go wrong.
- Practise, if it's something you can prepare for.
- Relax – go for a long walk, take a warm bath, listen to some calming music.

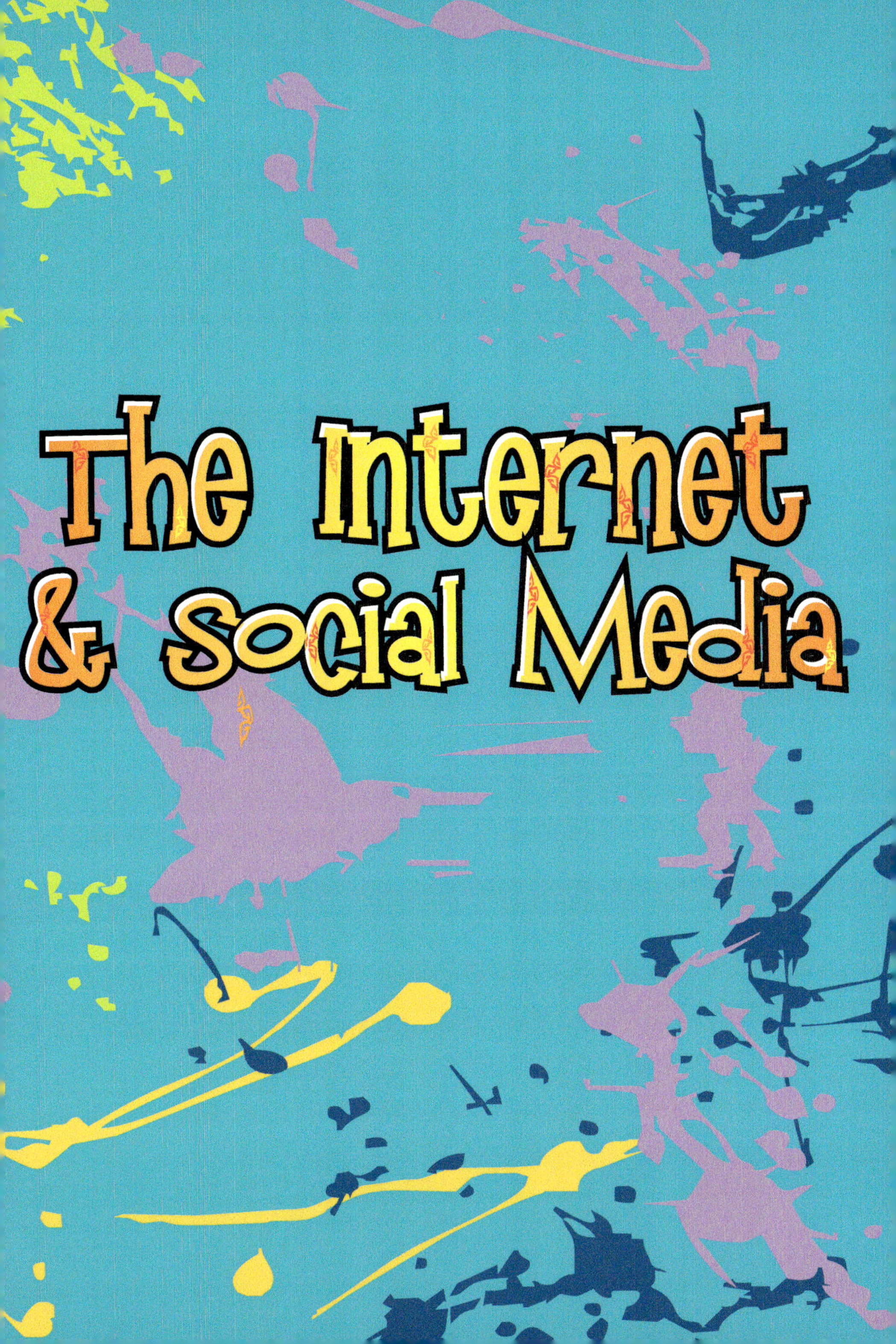
The Internet & Social Media

Social media and being safe online

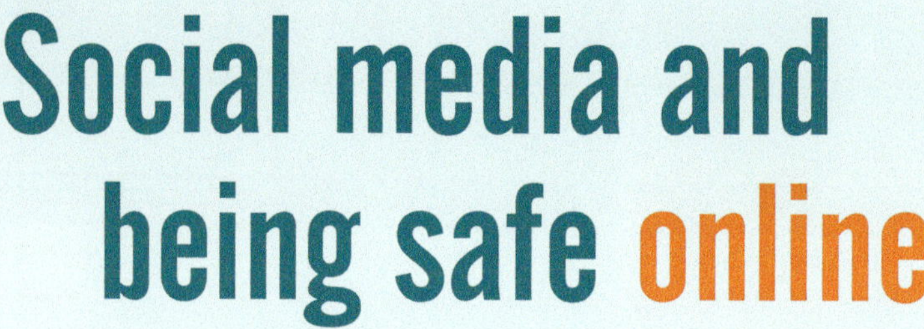

Whatever age you are right now, I am sure that you know all about the Internet, and may already use social media.

But did you know that you must reach a minimum age of 13 before you are legally able to have a social media account? There is GOOD reason for this.

Social media refers to online applications or Internet sites that allow you to share many aspects of your daily activities, thoughts and discoveries. From photographs to quotes, comments and interesting events with your mates – it can all be shared online.

The problem is that many kids allow lots of people to access their online profiles and make comments. They can also SHARE pictures that you post.

There is nothing wrong with having online friends, however you need to remember that your ONLINE WORLD is just as REAL as your REAL LIFE WORLD.

Everything that you post (put on your profile) and share can be SAVED and SHARED anywhere in the online world by any of your online friends.

A word of advice here: Don't allow just anyone to 'friend' you on Facebook, or follow you on Instagram or other social media accounts. You need to use these tools wisely.

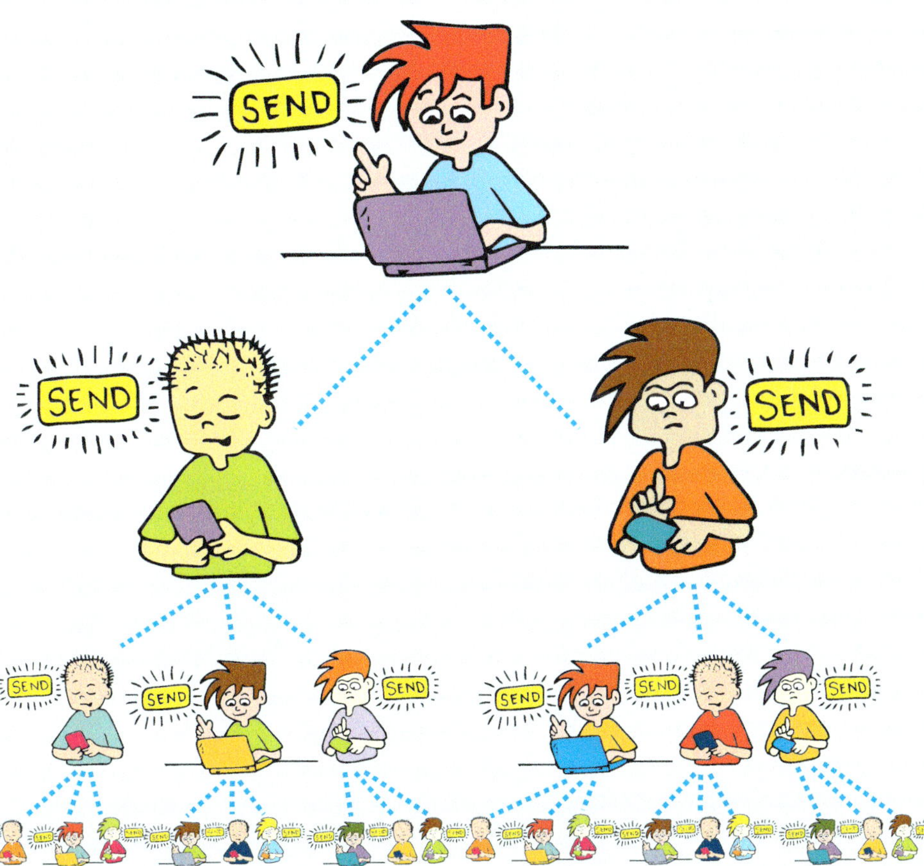

Guidelines for using social media

- Never post a picture/photograph that you would not be happy for ANYONE TO SEE.
- Take some time to THINK THROUGH what you want to say before you send a message or email. Sometimes, we need to put ourselves in another person's position to better understand how that person might respond.
- Never reveal PERSONAL DETAILS about yourself. For example, the school you attend or where you live.
- Do not tell anyone online what your phone number or address is because you have no way of ever knowing whether someone else online is ROLE-PLAYING – pretending to be someone he or she is not.
- Do not participate in any conversations that you would not normally be a part of 'IN REAL LIFE'. If you do not gossip about other people in person, do not do it online. It is exactly the same thing.

- If you do use an instant messaging service or app, choose only a small group of people you TRUST, and keep it to that.

- BE OPEN about what you are doing. Do not lock yourself away from your family and parents. If you cannot show your parents what you are saying, you may need to reconsider what you're saying.

- Before sending an SMS/message or commenting on social media, ask yourself the following simple question: 'Would I be happy SAYING this in person?'

- If you receive any threats or harassing messages on social media, do not instantly delete them. TELL **a trusted adult or parent straight away.** They can help you with the issue. Remember, nothing is SO BAD that they cannot help you through it.

More helpful information on Internet safety:

www.cybersmart.gov.au

Choose your influences

Imagine your mind as being like a great big SPONGE. Everything that you allow into your mind will be absorbed, just as a sponge absorbs liquid. Your mind cannot say, 'No, I choose not to absorb that image'. It does so anyway.

What do you want your mind to absorb?
Think about the programs you watch online or on television. What sort of messages are they sending to your mind? You have the power to choose what will influence you: movies, books, magazines, music, whatever you present to your mind.

Movies

It is a good idea to make a decision NOW regarding what sort of movies you will allow yourself to be exposed to. That way, you can make an easy choice if friends want to see or hire a certain type of movie.

Listen to your parents. They will give you good guidelines because they are looking out for your best interests.

Don't just go along with the crowd on this one. Remember to choose wisely.

Television programs

As with movies, you always have a CHOICE with the television remote control. If the programs that you watch do not meet with your measure of personal integrity – your morals and values – change the channel.

It is also important to remember that many television programs are based on fiction, not real life. Your mind subconsciously begins to believe that these programs reflect exactly what real life is. Many TV shows do not portray what real life is for the majority of the population, yet our thoughts and ideas may influence what we think should be a reality. Don't get fooled by this.

Online shows

It's the same principle with online shows and what you see on video sites. Make a decision about what's appropriate and what isn't. Stay away from videos and channels that don't match your personal values. Be proud of the decisions you make – they mark your character and set you apart as someone who won't compromise personal moral choices.

Music

Music is a powerful influence, probably one of the most significant in your life. Choose carefully the music that you allow into your mind. It is hard to erase the words and images once they enter your mind.

Music, however, can be a powerful and positive influence, too. It can help you relax and feel peaceful. Look at the LYRICS (words) to a song before you stream or buy music. That way, you can make a choice if you want to be influenced by the music and lyrics or not.

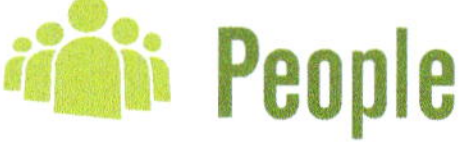

People

We always have a choice about connecting with the people we WANT to spend time with, and influence our thinking and behaviours.

You become like the people you hang out with for most of the time. If you choose to be friends with negative people or those who want to lead you into trouble, the chances are that you will start to become just like them. On the other hand, choosing to hang out with positive and happy people will influence you that way, too.

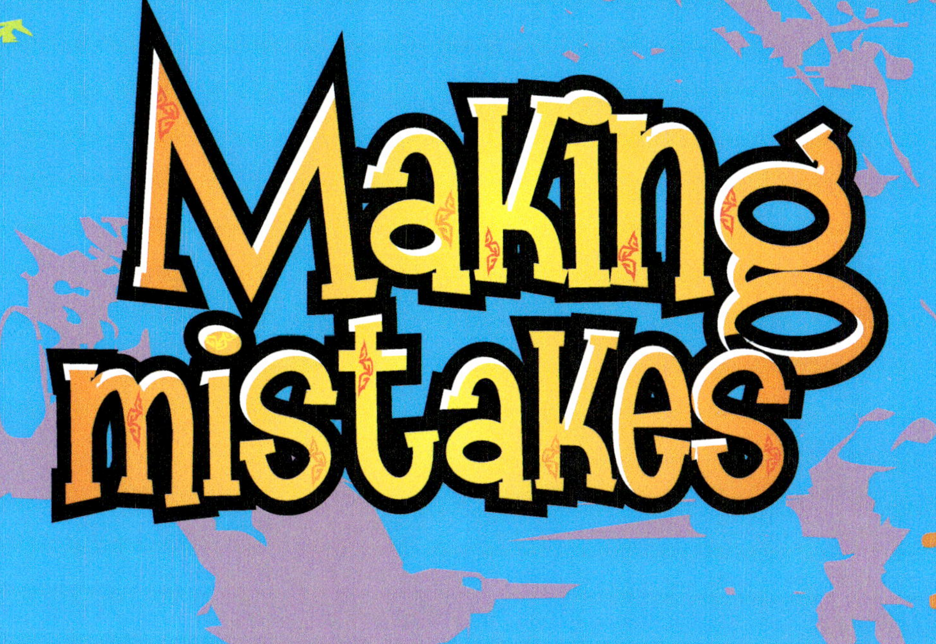
Making mistakes

Mistakes

Woops... Error... Booboo...

Have you ever made a mistake?
If you're anything like me, you've made LOADS of them. Making mistakes is a big part of life and learning.

It's something that we all need to accept will happen from time to time. The trick is to learn how to USE mistakes to your advantage.

Mistakes can be seen as an opportunity to GROW and MAKE CHANGES in how we behave and what decisions we make. You can look at the word mistake another way – MIS·TAKE – which actually means to try again; have another go.

When we make mistakes, we can feel:

— **Worried**
— **Sick in our stomach**
— **Nervous**
— **Sad**
— **Disappointed**
— **Angry**
— **Hopeless**
— **...and many other negative feelings.**

It's not fun when we make mistakes; however the lesson for all of us is to LEARN from them.

Just about any person you can think of throughout history has made mistakes. Even the most SUCCESSFUL and ACCOMPLISHED people have made plenty of mistakes along the way to reach their positions of success. So you're in great company.

THOMAS EDISON was a famous inventor who created the light globe. Historians suggest he may have got it wrong well over a thousand times before he finally got it right!

Perhaps you are given a spelling test at school. You might get words wrong. Don't worry – you now have a great opportunity to PRACTISE the words you misspelt and get them correct the next time.

Mistakes are only a problem if you DON'T learn from them!

Other famous people who didn't get it right the first time:
They learned from their mistakes and succeeded ultimately in achieving great successes.
*** Walt Disney**
*** Steve Jobs**
*** Abraham Lincoln**
*** Winston Churchill**

Your mistake

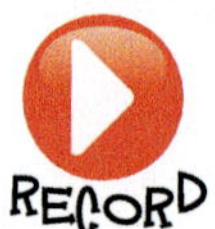

Write about a time when you made a mistake.
What happened?

The lesson

What did you learn from this mistake?
How will you do better next time?

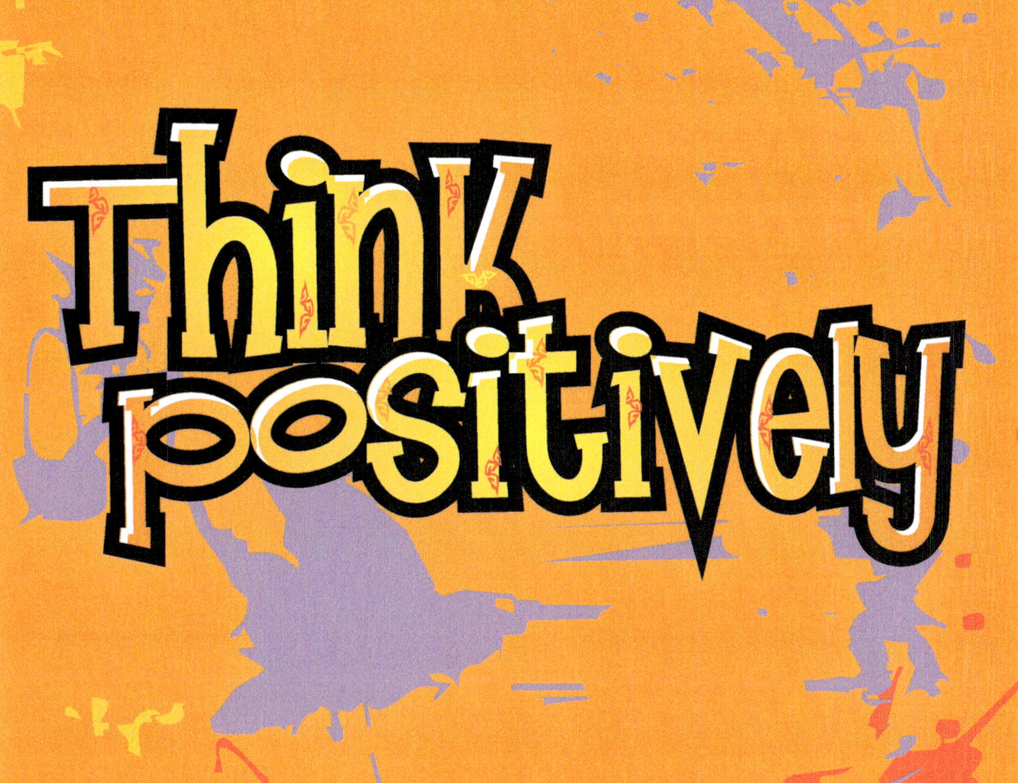
Think positively

Watching your words

Have you ever caught yourself saying things like:

> *'I'm **hopeless** at this.'*
> *'I can't get it right.'*
> *'I'm so **dumb**.'*
> *'I have **no friends**.'*
> *'No one likes me.'*
> *'I'm **ugly**, unlovable.'*

Think about this for a moment, would you actually walk up to someone and say:

> *'Nobody likes you,'* or
> *'You are **so** hopeless?'*

Of course, you probably wouldn't say these things to another person! Yet we often say such words to OURSELVES. Maybe we don't say these out loud, but even THINKING these things affects us.

When you tell yourself that you are a failure, hopeless, dumb or unlikeable, you are in fact, BULLYING YOURSELF!

God created you as a very cool and amazingly likeable person. Don't spend your time and energy speaking negatively about yourself.

Write a positive letter to yourself

Imagine that you have a mate who has been feeling really down and negative. He hasn't been happy or his usual self and is not participating in things that he usually enjoys doing.

Now, pretend that guy is YOU.

Write a letter to yourself, reminding you how amazing, smart and brave you are.

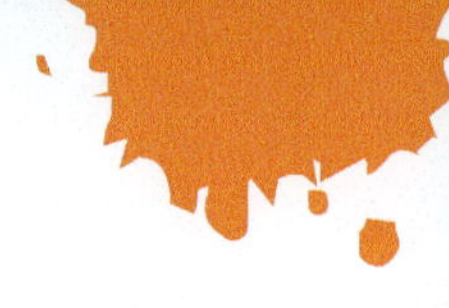

When difficult things happen...

Life is certainly not always easy.

No matter what age you are, STRUGGLES or TOUGH TIMES will occur every now and then.

You may experience struggles with your friendships, school, learning, family situations or illnesses. There are some experiences that we just cannot avoid, like getting a bad case of chicken pox that forces you to miss out on your basketball grand final.

Some struggles and difficult times are unavoidable, but we can always choose HOW we will respond to tough circumstances. We can also rely on other people – family and friends – to help us manage our way through those difficult times.

We can CHOOSE to let those tough experiences make us feel SAD, ANGRY or HURT, or we can learn to accept the challenging times and use them to make us STRONGER and WISER.

Sometimes...

Sometimes...	*life doesn't seem very fair.*
Sometimes...	*bad things just happen for no reason at all.*
Sometimes...	*we can feel really sad when things are different to how they once were.*
Sometimes...	*it's difficult to accept what life throws at us.*
Sometimes...	*we need to take a big, deep breath and let it be.*
Sometimes...	*we need to lean on other people for a time (that's OK though; they can lean on you sometime if needed).*
Sometimes...	*there will be valuable lessons we will learn along the way (even if it's a really tough experience).*
And quite often...	*you will come out through the end of this experience stronger, wiser and even better equipped to face future challenges.*

Sharon Witt

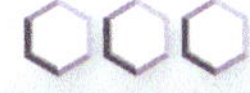

You CAN make a difference

The starfish story...

A young boy was standing on a beach surrounded by hundreds and perhaps thousands of tiny starfish that had washed up on the beach and were slowly dying.

A man some distance away observed the boy reaching down, picking up a starfish and throwing it back in the ocean. One at a time, he picked up a starfish and tossed it back in the sea.

As the man approached the boy, he stopped and asked a question.

'Boy, can't you see that there are literally thousands of starfish here washed up on the beach? They will surely die in this hot sun. Don't you understand that you cannot possibly ***make a difference?'***

The boy responded by reaching down, picking up another starfish and tossing it back in the ocean.

'Made a difference to ***that one!'*** *he replied.*

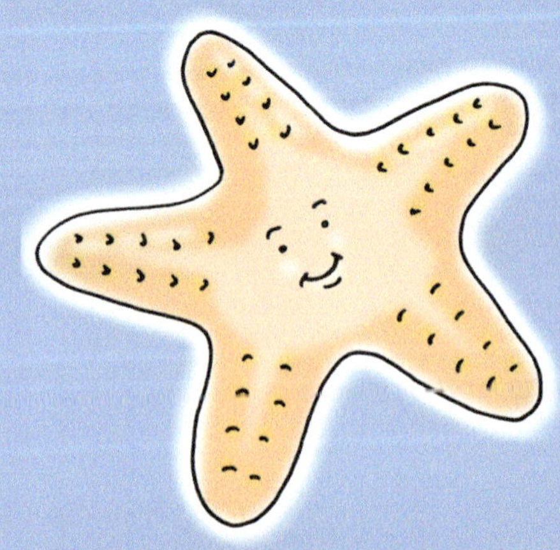

Have some perspective

It's not the end of the world!

Have you ever been working on a school project and accidentally spilt your drink all over it? I have!

You immediately go into major PANIC mode.
'Oh no. This is the end of the world!'
'My project is completely ruined.'
'I'm going to FAIL *school now and wind up* HOMELESS!*'*
Talk about overreacting!

We can totally lose PERSPECTIVE sometimes. In actual fact, we can wipe off most of the spilt drink, let it dry out and hand it to our teacher with some 'bonus' artwork, free of charge.

Sometimes, it can be difficult to keep things in perspective.

You might look at a situation such as ruining a school project as the end of the world, whereas your mum might come into the room and see that the situation as not nearly as desperate and drastic as you think. She wipes up the mess, places your project outside in the sunshine and reassures you that this is one of MANY mishaps that will happen in your lifetime. Her wise words to you are: 'It's not the end of the world'.

One day, our family was staying in a caravan park in a quiet country town. The park was very bushy and full of trees. A storm descended on the town, waking us in the middle of the night with the sound of an almighty CRASH – so loud it made our caravan SHAKE!

We went outside to investigate, only to see a GIANT tree had crashed down right next to us, completely covering the neighbouring car. In fact, we could only see the tree trunk, branches and leaves on top of the car.

The car was completely destroyed, and the couple next door could have been understandably distraught about losing their vehicle.

They had, however, a great perspective. They chose to feel relief, being thankful that the tree had fallen on to their replaceable car, and not THEM as they lay in their caravan, sound asleep.

All about perspective: do you see two faces or a vase?

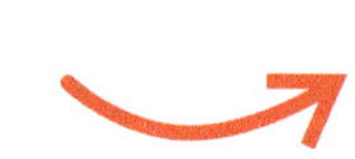

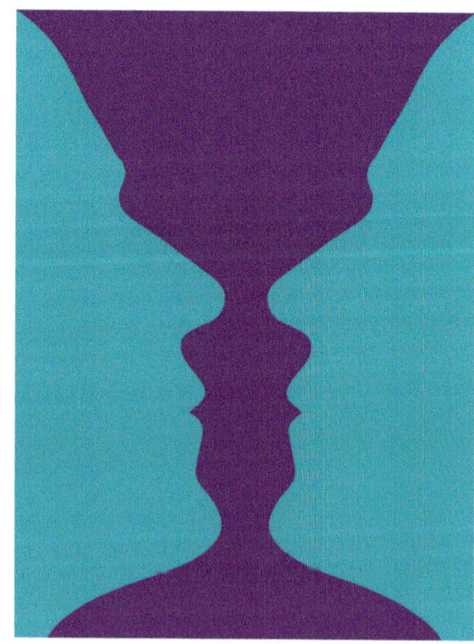

Take 5

When something happens that temporarily makes you think:

'Oh no! This is terrible.'

'I cannot cope.'

'This is a disaster!'

STOP! TAKE 5!

Take a DEEP BREATH and count to five in big, long and easy breaths and then take five minutes to see if there is a different way to look at the experience. See if you can grab hold of a different perspective. Sometimes, a good night's sleep will help. Or talk to a trusted friend or family member.

PRAY.

You will see the problem in a whole new light.

It may not be so bad after all.

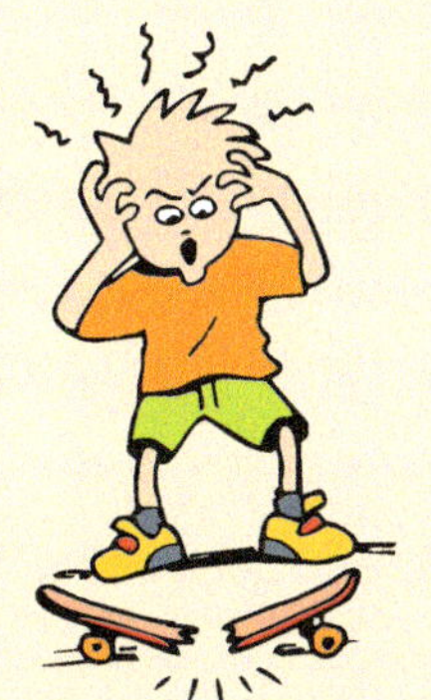

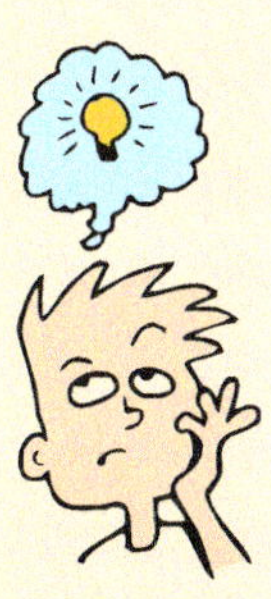

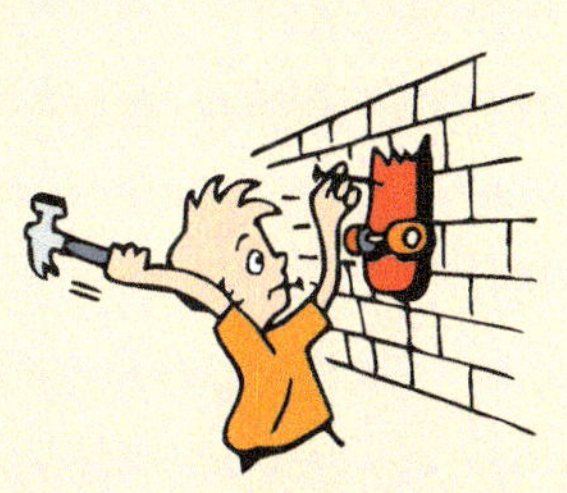

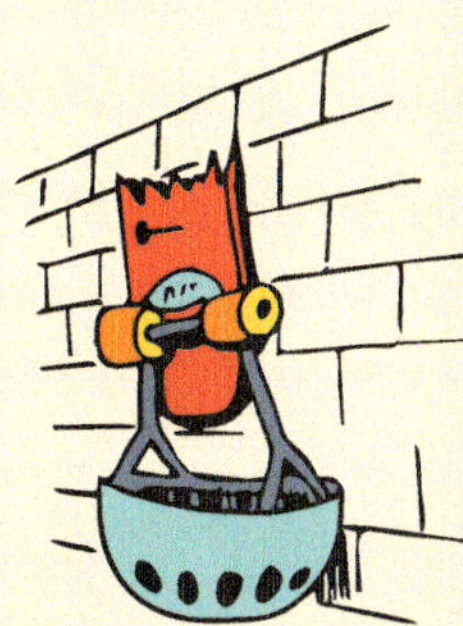

Your tongue: A sword?

Go for peacemaking, not destruction

You may be a person who occasionally calls people names.

You need to understand that the words that come out of your mouth can have a LASTING effect, even though you may not think so at the time.

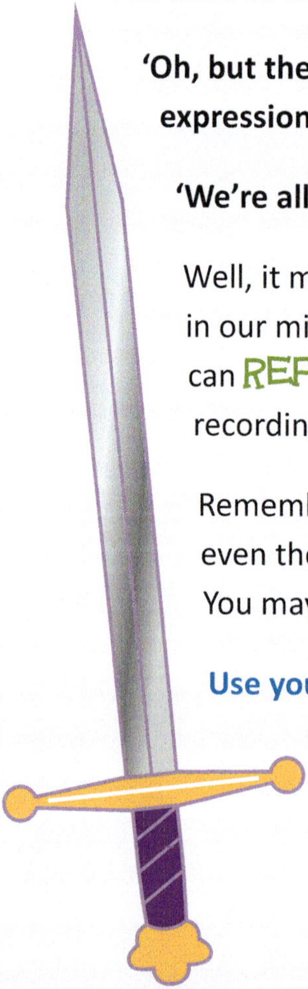

'Oh, but they know that I am only *joking*,' is a common expression people use to justify calling others names.

'We're all mates, aren't we?'

Well, it may seem so, but words have a way of sticking in our minds if they are offensive or hurtful. And they can REPLAY themselves over and over again like a recording in our minds for as long as we allow them to.

Remember that your tongue is a very powerful weapon, even though you may not physically hurt someone. You may cause even greater emotional damage.

Use your words to build another person up, not destroy his or her self-image.

Make your tongue a PEACEMAKER, not a destructive WEAPON.

Goals and dreams

We all have goals and dreams in life: Things that we would love to DO, ACHIEVE and BE.

When I was young, I wanted to be a famous singer and actress on television. I even practised my singing pose in front of the mirror! I wanted to travel the world and have everyone seek my autograph.

Then, as I grew older, I realised that I really enjoyed working with children (as well as acting) and decided I would become a teacher. After many more years, I soon discovered that I *loved* to write for young people. The very fact that you are reading this book *right now* is the result of one girl (*me*) having GOALS and DREAMS.

You have the SAME opportunities and the same amount of minutes in each day as everybody else!

No matter what age you are, write down your dreams and goals and **go for it.** Don't let ANYONE tell you that you can't achieve them or that they are silly.

Inside of you is great CREATIVITY, as well as IMAGINATION and lots of adventures to be had as you unwrap and discover your unique dreams and gifts.

Dream BIG

starting with the small goals

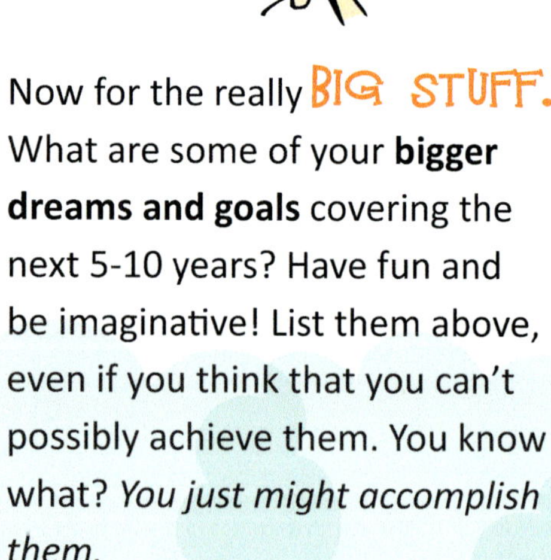

Start small. List above some of the SMALL DREAMS and goals that you would like to achieve in the near future – during the coming year.

Now for the really BIG STUFF. What are some of your **bigger dreams and goals** covering the next 5-10 years? Have fun and be imaginative! List them above, even if you think that you can't possibly achieve them. You know what? *You just might accomplish them.*

Think BIG, and follow your DREAMS

Don't let anyone tell you
That you cannot achieve
Your own hopes and dreams.
Within you is great hope, creativity and SPARK!
You can dream, create, inspire, achieve
Whatever is in your heart and imagination.
Inside of you are GREAT *gifts!*
Use your gifts to impact this world
Ignore those who tell you that you're
Too young
Or not talented enough to achieve your dreams
Read, investigate, plan and inspire yourself
To follow your DREAMS!
YOU *are* GIFTED
YOU *are* AMAZING
YOU *are* BLESSED
You are a GIFT *to this world!*

Sharon Witt

Yay! You've done it!

But there's more to life after you finish this page.

I am ***so*** happy that you have made it through WISEGUYS! I really hope and pray that you have gained some practical advice and help in how to handle some of life's challenges and how you can be all that you were created to be.

Always remember that inside of you is great wisdom, as well as strength and courage. Believe me, you will go far.

There is a **heap of help** out there for the problems and battles you will face along the way. Remember to ask your friends and trusted adults... and pray to God to guide you through life and make wise decisions.

You are going to make a HUGE difference in this world, just because YOU are in it!

Sharon

Notes, credits, sources

1. Minecraft online link: https://minecraft.net
2. Biscuiting is also known as tubing: http://tinyurl.com/ohfjabm
3. Archbishop Desmond Tutu foundation biography: http://tinyurl.com/9jqoec
4. Movie actor profile: http://tinyurl.com/kne8zg
5. German philosopher profile: http://tinyurl.com/dkbt9g
6. Permission granted for use of passage.
7. Permission granted for use of passage.
8. Publisher's website for C S Lewis.
9. American writer and artist who died in 1915.

Notes

Notes